INTRODUCTION TO INSECT PEST MANAGEMENT
Robert L. Metcalf and William H. Luckman, Editors

OUR ACOUSTIC ENVIRONMENT
Frederick A. White

ENVIRONMENTAL DATA HANDLING
George B. Heaslip

THE MEASUREMENT OF AIRBORNE PARTICLES
Richard D. Cadle

ANALYSIS OF AIR POLLUTANTS
Peter O. Warner

ENVIRONMENTAL INDICES
Herbert Inhaber

URBAN COSTS OF CLIMATE MODIFICATION
Terry A. Ferrar, Editor

CHEMICAL CONTROL OF INSECT BEHAVIOR: THEORY AND APPLICATION
H. H. Shorey and John J. McKelvey, Jr.

MERCURY CONTAMINATION: A HUMAN TRAGEDY
Patricia A. D'Itri and Frank M. D'Itri

POLLUTANTS AND HIGH RISK GROUPS
Edward J. Calabrese

SULFUR IN THE ENVIRONMENT, Parts I and II
Jerome O. Nriagu, Editor

FOOD, CLIMATE, AND MAN
Margaret R. Biswas and Asit K. Biswas, Editors

ENERGY UTILIZATION AND ENVIRONMENTAL HEALTH: METHODS FOR PREDICTION AND EVALUATION OF IMPACT ON HUMAN HEALTH
Richard A. Wadden, Editor

RESOURCE RECOVERY AND RECYCLING
A. F. M. Barton

ENERGY UTILIZATION AND ENVIRONMENTAL HEALTH

ENERGY UTILIZATION AND ENVIRONMENTAL HEALTH

METHODS FOR PREDICTION AND EVALUATION OF IMPACT ON HUMAN HEALTH

EDITED BY

RICHARD A. WADDEN

ENVIRONMENTAL HEALTH SCIENCES
SCHOOL OF PUBLIC HEALTH
UNIVERSITY OF ILLINOIS
CHICAGO, ILLINOIS

A WILEY-INTERSCIENCE PUBLICATION

JOHN WILEY & SONS

NEW YORK • CHICHESTER • BRISBANE • TORONTO

Library of Congress Cataloging in Publication Data

Main entry under title:
Energy utilization and environmental health.

(Environmental science and technology)
"A Wiley-Interscience publication."
Includes index.
1. Environmental health—Evaluation. 2. Environmental impact analysis. 3. Power resources—Hygienic aspects. I. Wadden, R. A.

RA566.E43 614.7 78-9688
ISBN 0-471-04185-8

Printed in the United States of America

10 9 8 7 6 5 4 3 2 1

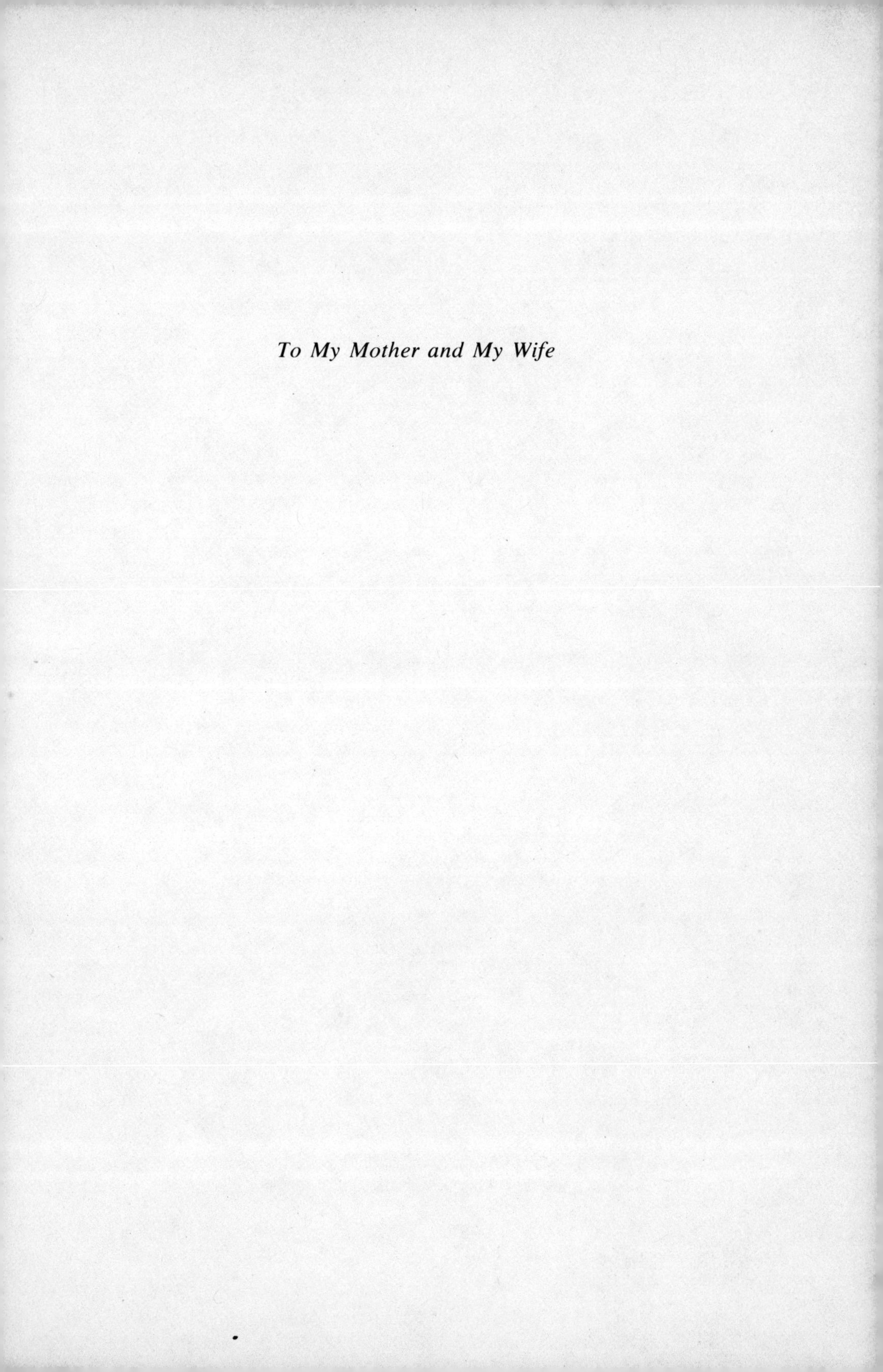

To My Mother and My Wife

CONTRIBUTORS

Robert J. Allen, Environmental Health Sciences
University of Illinois, School of Public Health

Lyndon R. Babcock, Jr., Environmental Health Sciences
University of Illinois School of Public Health

Gary R. Brenniman, Environmental Health Sciences
University of Illinois, School of Public Health

Bertram W. Carnow, Occupational and Environmental Medicine
University of Illinois, School of Public Health

Donna O. Farley, Suburban Cook County-Du Page
County Health Systems Agency, Oak Park, Illinois

William H. Hallenbeck, Environmental Health Sciences
University of Illinois, School of Public Health

Richard G. Hankett, Research and Development Division
Chicago Department of Public Works

Janet A. Holden, Environmental Health Sciences
University of Illinois, School of Public Health

Sally J. Jansen, Occupational and Environmental Medicine
University of Illinois, School of Public Health

William H. Kojola, Occupational and Environmental Medicine
University of Illinois, School of Public Health

Edward J. Koval
5018 South Laramie, Chicago, Illinois

Alvin L. Miller, Occupational and Environmental Medicine
University of Illinois, School of Public Health

Niren L. Nagda, Geomet Inc.
Gaithersburg, Maryland

Anneke de Werk Neal, Epidemiology
University of Illinois, School of Public Health

Peter A. Scheff, Environmental Health Sciences
University of Illinois, School of Public Health

Richard A. Wadden, Environmental Health Sciences
University of Illinois, School of Public Health

Arthur H. Wolff, Environmental Health Sciences
University of Illinois, School of Public Health

SERIES PREFACE

Environmental Science and Technology

The Environmental Science and Technology Series of Monographs, Textbooks, and Advances is devoted to the study of the quality of the environment and to the technology of its conservation. Environmental science therefore relates to the chemical, physical, and biological changes in the environment through contamination or modification, to the physical nature and biological behavior of air, water, soil, food, and waste as they are affected by man's agricultural, industrial, and social activities, and to the application of science and technology to the control and improvement of environmental quality.

The deterioration of environmental quality, which began when man first collected into villages and utilized fire, has existed as a serious problem under the ever-increasing impacts of exponentially increasing population and of industrializing society. Environmental contamination of air, water, soil, and food has become a threat to the continued existence of many plant and animal communities of the ecosystem and may ultimately threaten the very survival of the human race.

It seems clear that if we are to preserve for future generations some semblance of the biological order of the world of the past and hope to improve on the deteriorating standards of urban public health, environmental science and technology must quickly come to play a dominant role in designing our social and industrial structure for tomorrow. Scientifically rigorous criteria of environmental quality must be developed. Based in part on these criteria, realistic standards must be established and our technological progress must be tailored to meet them. It is obvious that civilization will continue to require increasing amounts of fuel, transportation, industrial chemicals, fertilizers, pesticides, and countless other products; and that it will continue to produce waste products of all descriptions. What is urgently needed is a total systems approach to modern civilization through which the pooled talents of scientists and engineers, in cooperation with social scientists and the medical profession, can be focused on the development of order and equilibrium in the presently disparate segments of the human environment. Most of the skills and tools that are needed are already in existence. We surely have a right to hope a technology that has created such manifold environmental problems is also capable of solving them. It is our hope that this Series in Environmental Sciences and Technology will not only serve to make this challenge more explicit to the established professionals, but that it also will help to stimulate the student toward the career opportunities in this vital area.

Robert L. Metcalf
James N. Pitts, Jr.
Werner Stumm

PREFACE

The production, distribution, and use of energy is a process basic to an industrial society. A variety of socioeconomic criteria must be considered when choosing how we are to best utilize our energy resources. Of great significance in such considerations is the prediction and evaluation of existing and potential human health effects due to energy sources and usage. Indeed, adverse health impact should exercise veto power over other criteria if construction or operation of energy facilities produces a nonviable environment.

Despite its importance, little attention has been given to health questions in site planning of energy production facilities or pollution control strategies. There have been only limited efforts toward prediction of the environmental health impact of pollutants on populations who may be exposed to such materials. Also of considerable concern is the advent of new processes and technologies for energy production which have their own unique pollution potential.

The purpose of this book is to explain and demonstrate evaluation methods that can be used to incorporate public health considerations into the planning process. The opening chapter (Sources, Receptors, and the Environment) outlines the role of these three major components, and their interrelationship, in the evaluation of environmental impact. Chapters 2 and 3 discuss receptor characterization, particularly emphasizing methods to identify, enumerate, and locate hypersusceptible populations, that is, those individuals who are likely to be first and most affected by pollution exposure. Chapters 4–6 report on several methods for quantitating the biological effects of environmental stress in humans. Characterization of environmental hazards in terms of quantitation and dispersal is covered in Chapters 7–9. The final four chapters show how these basic data and methods can be applied to real problems in environmental planning. The evaluations are carried out in considerable detail in an attempt to give the reader a practical grasp of how to go about quantitating the potential health ramifications of energy processes.

It is recognized that there are many deficiencies in our understanding of the cause and effect relationship between environmentally discharged pollutants and human health effects. But it is incumbent upon us as planners and scientists to use available information to make the best estimate possible, recognizing that such an estimate must be understood within the limitations of the supporting data, and that continual revision and updating will be a fact of life. We believe that the methods described here will be helpful for all who are concerned with the evaluation of environmental impact. We also hope that publication of these methods will stimulate others to develop even more meaningful measures of human health response to environmental stressors.

The development of this book was supported in part by a grant (G007602055) from the Office of Environmental Education, U.S. Office of Education, U.S. Department of Health, Education, and Welfare whose support is hereby acknowledged. Mr. Alfred Rosenbloom aided greatly with format, and his assistance was much appreciated. Most particularly, great thanks are due to Mrs. Vera Donlan and Ms. Lucille Vaughn for typing of the many drafts before the final manuscript was complete. I also wish to thank all those members of the University of Illinois School of Public Health who contributed in formal and nonformal ways to the final version of the book.

RICHARD A. WADDEN

Chicago, Illinois
May 1978

CONTENTS

ENERGY UTILIZATION AND ENVIRONMENTAL HEALTH

1

SOURCES, RECEPTORS, AND THE ENVIRONMENT

Richard A. Wadden

The present American life-style requires use of considerable amounts of air, water, energy, and mineral resources. On a per capita basis Americans use 30 times as much coal, 40 times as much crude steel, 60 times as much refined copper, and 80 times as much primary aluminum as are used in underdeveloped countries (1). How these resources are maintained or destroyed, dissipated or conserved, depleted or restored have significant implications for human health. How our societal needs can be provided for without harming ourselves is a legitimate requirement of the planning process.

Perception of the societal worth of a given project depends on comparison of the project's characteristics with one or more criteria that an individual, or groups of individuals, consider to be important. Projects that require such evaluation include those to do with transportation (shopping centers, highway networks, airports) and with energy production and use (nuclear and fossil fuel power plants, fusion and solar power, coal and oil conversion processes). Criteria that are often considered in the planning process are utility, accessibility, efficiency, and job and profit potential. Criteria that are rarely or cursorily applied include inconvenience to nonusers, degradation of natural resources to nonvaluable end products (such as the use of natural gas to produce carbon black), pollution potential, and most significantly, risk to human health.

While all the above factors, as well as others appropriate to a specific project, should be taken into account, the impact on human health should have effective veto power over all the rest. Establishment of a nonviable environment is self-defeating for any project. This discussion outlines an organized approach to evaluating the human health implications of projects that have the potential for release of hazardous materials into the environment.

To put in perspective the interaction of hazardous discharges with human health it is helpful to consider the relationships represented in Figures 1.1 and 1.2. Pollutants are discharged from pollutant sources. These discharges are commonly called emissions if they enter the air environment and effluents if entering the water environment. The amounts of emissions and effluents are best described by using a mass/time rate, such as pounds per hour or tons per day. As pollutants are released they are immediately mixed with whatever materials already exist in the air or water (baseline concentrations). In addition, they undergo chemical and physical changes both because of their interaction

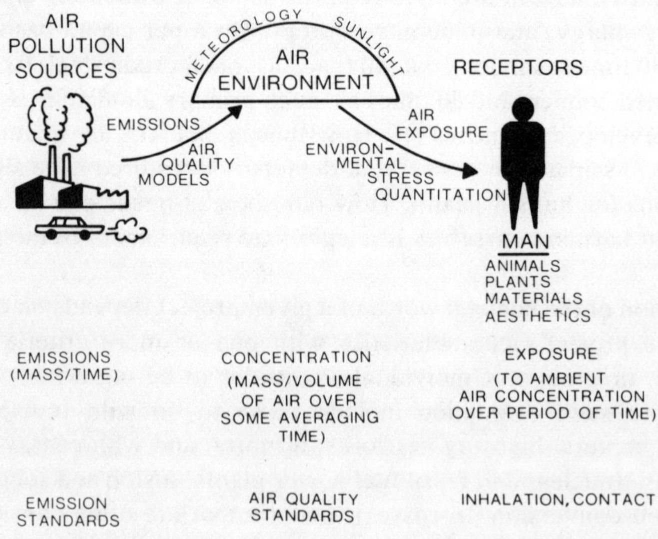

Figure 1.1. Sources, receptors, and the air environment.

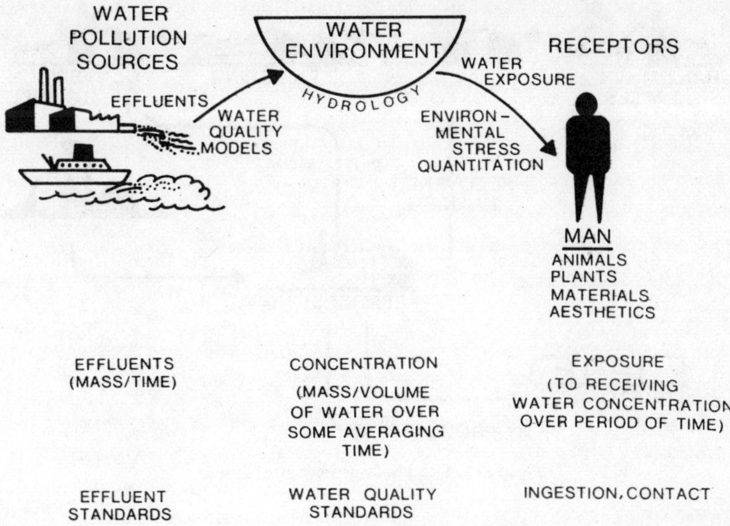

Figure 1.2. Sources, receptors, and the water environment.

with other pollutants, and because of the nature of the receiving air or water. For air, solar radiation and meteorologic effects, such as temperature inversions and windspeed, are important. For water, hydrologic considerations affect the dissipation or concentration of a pollutant.

Pollutants in air (or water) environments are characterized by measuring their mass per unit volume of air (or water), that is, their concentration. This concentration is related to a particular averaging time, which corresponds to the time interval of sample collection, or the time over which a number of samples are combined. The relationship between source emissions or effluents and environmental concentrations can be estimated by using air quality or water quality models.

The most important consideration of air and water pollution is the consequences that their environmental concentrations may have for human receptors. The relevant steps in evaluating such consequences require asking the following questions: What individuals are most at risk to the expected environmental hazards? How many of them are there? Where are they located with respect to the pollution source? How much are they likely to be affected by the additional environmental stress?

The consideration of all the factors noted above should be incorporated into the environmental impact analysis of a new energy source or use.

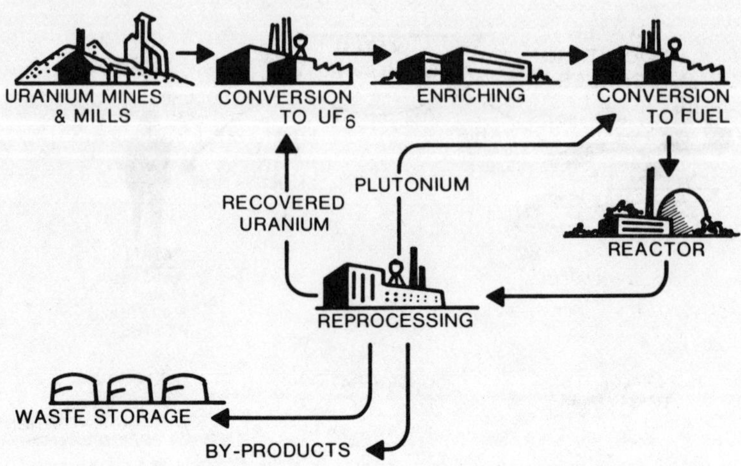

Figure 1.3. The nuclear fuel cycle.

Such an analysis may cover only a specific source and site evaluation with limited geographical considerations, or it may involve an evaluation of a total energy cycle. Figure 1.3 indicates such a cycle for nuclear fuel. The series of steps shown in Figure 1.3 is actually spread out over a large area (nationwide in the United States) and involves many complex processes at each location. At each step there are pollution and health consequences to be considered. Our focus throughout this book is mainly on health implications of specific sources or planning alternatives. However, the same procedures can also be applied to the steps of an energy cycle.

To summarize briefly then, the major steps in the overall review process (2) are:

1. Identification of hazards—raw material, type of process, method of operation.
2. Quantitation of hazardous wastes and byproducts—air, water, and soil.
3. Measurement of "baseline" conditions of the environment—present air, water, and soil quality.
4. Dispersion of hazardous discharges—what and how much goes where.
5. Identification, enumeration, and location of populations at risk.
6. Estimation of exposure levels and related health effects.

Each of these categories is discussed more completely in later chapters. It is important that the items listed above become a regular consideration for those planning and deciding upon projects with pollution potential. In addition, such considerations should be more specifically incorporated into legislation and regulations involving pollution sources. Finally, public agencies should be encouraged to investigate and follow up the health implications of existing and new projects that discharge environmental hazards. Our concern for material prosperity should not cause us to neglect our responsibilities for human health.

REFERENCES

1. Masters, G. M. *Introduction to Environmental Science and Technology.* John Wiley & Sons, New York, 1974.
2. Wadden, R. A. Health considerations in environmental planning. *Urban Planning and Development Div.,* ASCE **103**:27–37, 1977.

[illegible] plating and finishing [illegible] [illegible]
[illegible]
[illegible]
[illegible]
[illegible]
[illegible]
models. [illegible] Cadmium [illegible]

REFERENCES

1. [illegible]
2. [illegible]

RECEPTOR CHARACTERIZATION

2

IDENTIFICATION OF HYPERSUSCEPTIBLE POPULATIONS

Bertram W. Carnow

Some pollution accompanies any energy production and use. Therefore, the selection of energy sources and uses must be considered with care. To assess the options rationally, health cost of a particular energy source must be ascertained, and to do this a number of critical questions must be answered. How many people are adversely affected by respective energy sources? What is the range of physiological effects? Who in the population are most vulnerable? What might be the additional adverse effects of an increase in pollutants produced by a proposed change in methods or levels of energy production? If we approach intolerable levels of environmental contamination, how do we assess priorities for the generation and uses of energy?

To answer these questions it is first necessary to understand some basic concepts of environmental interactions with human populations. Humans, as biological organisms with varying degrees of resistance and adaptive capacity, are in continuous struggle to control the environment or to adapt to it. Any factor in the environment that increases its hostility, or anything lowering human resistance, decreases adaptability. For example, it is expected that the effect of irritation from toxic gases is strongest on those with inadequate cardiac or pulmonary reserve. Consequently those with adaptive capacity weakened by serious lung disease, heart disease, asthma, or other advanced chronic diseases have been the usual subjects of studies of the effects of air pollutants on humans (1–9). These studies suggest that frequency of cardiac and respiratory illness and death is associated with pollution levels. A simplified representation of the effect on the health continuum of a disturbance in the balance between adaptive capacity and environmental stress appears in Figure 2.1. Tables 2.1 and 2.2 list many of the factors that have been found, or might be expected, to increase susceptibility at levels that apparently do not affect healthy individuals. Several factors affect the sensitivity of a population. One set of risks inherent in the individual includes age, sex, general state of health, genetic predisposition, and preexisting disease. Another set relates to activity or place. Certain occupations present characteristic hazards. Other risks are characteristic of typical habitats. Locations and activities, including personal habits such as cigarette smoking or eating patterns, frequently reflect an economic status with a high risk of disease.

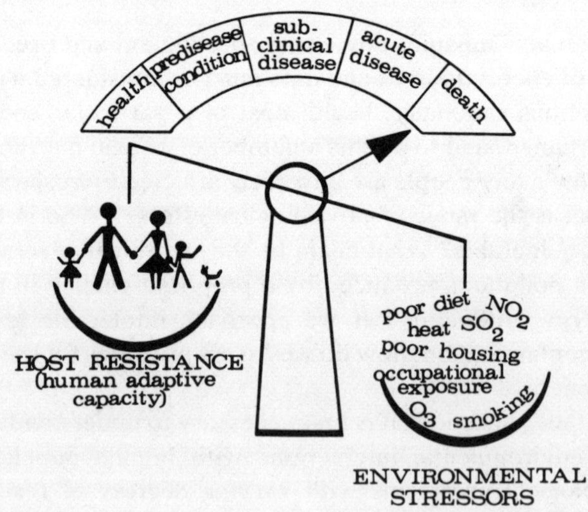

Figure 2.1. Environmental stressors in the public health continuum.

Table 2.1 Populations at High Risk to Environmental Pollutants because of Cardiac Deficiencies

Genetically Deficient

[a]Hypercholesterolemia
[a]Diabetes with atherosclerosis

Congenital Disease

[a]Tetralogy of fallot
[a]Atrial or ventricular wall defects
[a]Valvular defects

Chronic Disease

Cor pulmonale (secondary to chronic obstructive pulmonary disease)
Hypertension with left ventricular disease
Coronary insufficiency ([a]with or without angina)
Rheumatic heart disease
[a]Congestive heart failure (secondary to atherosclerotic heart disease)

Other Environmental Factors

Cigarette smoking
[a]Heavy work exposure

[a] No data—but might be expected to be at high risk.

Those hypersusceptible to stress are a large segment of the U.S. population. Specifically they include: (1) inhabitants of congested urban areas typified by psychosocial tension, poor nutrition, overcrowding, inadequate heating, and other factors associated with poverty; (2) fetuses, neonates, and preschool children; (3) the geriatric population whose medical history includes a high frequency of cardiovascular and cardiopulmonary disease; (4) those suffering from advanced bronchitis, emphysema, asthma, or other diseases whose symptoms worsen upon exposure to polluted air; (5) cigarette smokers and those exposed to large amounts of cigarette smoke, especially individuals already sustaining a body burden of a variety of noxious gases and particulate matter; (6) those involved in very heavy physical exertion requiring optimal energy transport; (7) people exposed by occupation or habitat to hazardous stresses, such as

Table 2.2 Populations at High Risk to Environmental Pollutants because of Pulmonary Deficiencies

Genetically Deficient

Asthma
Cystic fibrosis
Alpha antitrypsin deficiency
Cystic disease of lung

Chronic Disease

Chronic bronchitis
Emphysema
[a]Kyphoscoliosis
[a]Advanced (active or inactive) tuberculosis, histoplasmosis
[a]Bronchiectasis

Other Environmental Factors

Cigarette smokers
Workers exposed to dusts, fumes, smokes, aerosols, gases

Others

[a]Prematures
[a]Newborns
Preschool children
The poor, and those exposed to other environmental stresses such as overcrowding, malnutrition, poor heating
[a]Obesity

[a] No data—but might be expected to be at high risk.

asbestos, beryllium, or cotton dust, which may lead to diffuse scarring, fibrosis, and reduced elasticity of the lungs; (8) those with genetic handicaps such as asthma, alpha-l-antitrypsin deficiency or cystic fibrosis.

Figure 2.2 is an idealized representation of population responses to environmental stressors. As the degree of stress increases, that is, the burden of pollution, the severity of the effects (or the population affected) increases. A given level of stress will have different effects on given subpopulations. For example, pollution level x in the figure may cause the death of those most at risk, the aged with advanced cardiac and pulmo-

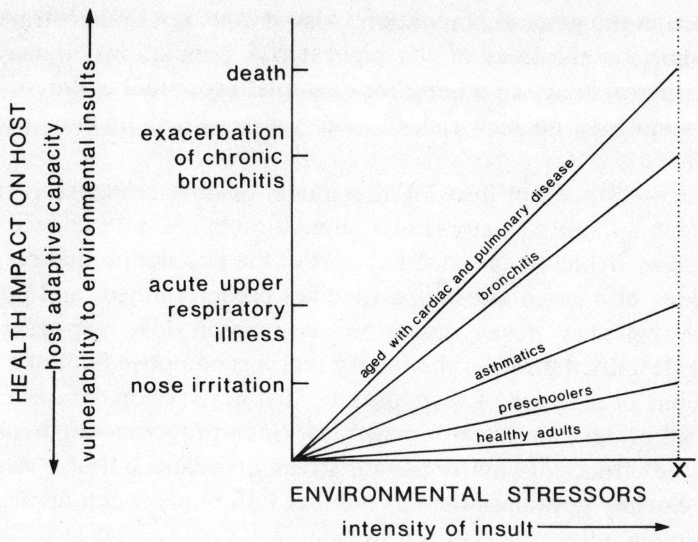

Figure 2.2. Population response to environmental stressors.

nary diseases; it might exacerbate chronic bronchitis; cause upper respiratory infections; increase the numbers and frequency of asthmatic attacks; or increase nose or sinus irritation in preschool children. Healthy adults would not be affected perceptibly by level x. (However, it should be recognized that the effects of long-time exposure to low levels, even on the healthy, have not been adequately documented.)

Figure 2.2 is, of course, merely schematic. Conceptually it applies to any specific environmental stressor. For air pollutants such as sulfur dioxide the population at highest risk would be the aged with cardiac and respiratory disease. For water viruses those at high risk might include very young children and those with liver disease who might be highly susceptible to hepatitis virus. Clues to whom should be considered may be derived from examining the organ or organs most likely to be stressed by the pollutants, and then defining in the general population those groups with poor adaptive capacity of this organ. If we consider the liver in this regard, hypersusceptible groups include those with alcoholism, individuals with fatty livers due to malnutrition, and those whose livers have undergone inflammatory changes due to heavy exposure to carbon tetrachloride or other similar solvents.

The diagram does not weight the subpopulations according to their distribution in the general population. Also it does not demonstrate that, while x shortens the lives of the highest risk populations, it may also decrease the resistance of others, for example, preschool children, to the end that some will be high risk in later years with their lives possibly shortened.

The concept we adopt in using this model of dose-response is that in general the response to a stress in a population is not pure chance but is determined by definable factors. The part of the population that responds to low doses of a given stress is a specific, predetermined, and possibly identifiable category. Even though the population dose-response curve cannot be described exactly, the theory that it is composed not of a single response but of a series of responses by distinct subpopulations can be quite useful in designing health programs. Such programs must consider not only the effects of environmental stress on health but also whom is affected. Society appraises the same effect differently when applied to a child, a young adult, or a retired person.

The physical and biological sciences are able to contribute to estimates of the bioenvironment's basic effects on public health. The social sciences assist in assigning values to specific effects on subpopulations. Society as a whole, however, decides how to use such information. It must be emphasized that the concept of a threshold effect exemplified by defining "safe levels" for a heterogeneous population has made it impossible over the years to quantitate populations at risk. It implies a "safe for everyone" level below this number and an "unsafe for anyone" level above this number. Rejection of this concept makes it possible to begin to define variations in risk at every level of pollution. There may be a safe level in a sense that effect may never be measurable. At virtually every level of stress, however, some die, some may fall ill, and some suffer minor insults depending on individual capacity to adapt.

Certain environmental effects have yet to be shown to lead to chronic or progressive disease, although their effects on individuals warrant attentive monitoring. Examples of these include elevated carboxyhemoglobin levels in smokers and urban dwellers, decreased respiratory function in children in highly populated areas, and lower antibody titers and influence of viruses among smokers compared to nonsmokers. Procedures that measure change in the small peripheral airways are now being used to evaluate pollutant effects on lungs. These procedures indicate that small airways are affected early and at levels of pollution much lower than were previously thought to be of concern. Earlier evaluation methods considered only large airways and concluded that no health effect occurred at these levels.

Figure 2.2 points up the need for recognizing health and disease as a continuum and not as sharply defined entities. The World Health Organization's definition of health (10), ". . . not only the absence of disease but a state of physical and mental well-being . . ." is hardly achievable in an urban center with all of its physical irritants, emotional stress, noise, and other similar stressors. The long incubation periods for most environmentally related diseases, including chronic pulmonary disease and cancer, point up the need to focus on preclinical factors and subclinical disease.

REFERENCES

1. Aronow, W. A. and Isbell, M. W. Carbon monoxide effect on exercise-induced angina pectoris. *Ann. Intern. Med.* **79**:392–395, 1973.
2. Carnow, B. W. and Meier, P. Air pollution and pulmonary cancer. *Arch. Environ. Health* **27**:207–218, 1973.
3. National Academy of Sciences. *Proceedings of the Conference on Health Effects of Air Pollutants*. U.S. Government Printing Office, No. 93-15, Washington, DC, 1973.
4. U.S. Department of Health, Education, and Welfare. *Air Quality Criteria for Carbon Monoxide*, AP-62, U.S. Government Printing Office, Washington, DC, 1970.
5. U.S. Department of Health, Education, and Welfare. *Air Quality Criteria for Nitrogen Oxides*, AP-84, U.S. Government Printing Office, Washington, DC, 1971.
6. U.S. Department of Health, Education, and Welfare. *Air Quality Criteria for Particulate Matter*, AP-49, U.S. Government Printing Office, Washington, DC, 1969.
7. U.S. Department of Health, Education, and Welfare. *Air Quality Criteria for Photochemical Oxidants*, AP-63, U.S. Government Printing Office, Washington, DC, 1970
8. U.S. Department of Health, Education, and Welfare. *Air Quality Criteria for Sulfur Oxides*, AP-50, U.S. Government Printing Office, Washington, DC, 1969.
9. U.S. Environmental Protection Agency. *Health Consequences of Sulfur Oxides: A Report from CHESS 1970–71*. EPA Report No. 650/1-74-004, Research Triangle Park, NC, 1974.
10. World Health Organization. *Health Hazards of the Human Environment*. United Nations, 1972.

[illegible]

[illegible]

[illegible]

1. [illegible]

2. [illegible]

3. [illegible]

4. [illegible]

5. [illegible]

6. [illegible] Government Printing Office, Washington [illegible]

7. [illegible] Washington [illegible]

8. [illegible] Government Printing Office, Washington, D.C. [illegible]

9. [illegible]

10. [illegible]

3

ENUMERATION AND LOCATION OF HYPERSUSCEPTIBLE POPULATIONS

Donna O. Farley

In order to estimate health impacts of environmental pollutant sources, the population groups most susceptible to the pollutants emitted must be identified, enumerated, and located relative to the sources. Potential health effects can be estimated by combining: (1) the numbers of high risk persons exposed, (2) the levels of pollutant exposure received, and (3) a measure of physiological response to that exposure.

Within any given area, population densities will not be uniform. The more precisely the distribution of each hypersusceptible population can be quantified, the more accurately the health impacts of pollutants within an area can be predicted. A frequently used procedure is to divide an area of interest into subareas, thereby providing a geographical grid within which high-risk populations can be enumerated. Since groups that are selected for enumeration must be quantifiable for these areas and subareas, the availability of data at the relevant geographical scale must be assessed. The applicability of enumeration techniques to that scale must also be determined.

Techniques for enumerating hypersusceptible populations fall into three categories that depend on how hypersusceptibility is characterized. One or more of these techniques may be used to estimate the size of various populations included in a health impact analysis.

DEMOGRAPHIC CHARACTERISTICS

This technique enumerates persons whose hypersusceptibility can be defined by demographic characteristics such as youth or old age. The primary sources of data are the U.S. Bureau of the Census (1) or state census data. Both the U.S. Decennial Census and national population estimates for intermediate years provide data on the total population for limited geographical areas. Characteristics of the population such as age, race, or income are also available in printed census reports or on computer tapes.

The census data are available by blocks, census tracts, or enumeration districts. These units, however, have geographical boundaries unique to the census. Either their boundaries must be used for subareas, or census data must be translated to the grid system being used. Extensive translation will require a computer and probably access to census data stored on tape rather than in published reports.

FACILITIES OCCUPIED BY HYPERSUSCEPTIBLE POPULATIONS

Among the facilities included in this category are acute-care hospitals, long-term care facilities, day-care centers, and schools. Because data must be expressed as the number of hypersusceptible persons in each subarea, a detailed listing must be made of all facilities, including their exact locations and capacities for occupancy. The capacity (or actual average occupancy, if available) of each facility is then assigned to the subarea in which the facility is located. See references (2,3) for examples of use of the method.

Because of their very specific site locations, high-risk facilities can be used to enumerate hypersusceptible populations on virtually any geographic scale. Unlike census information however, these data do not necessarily represent persons living at the facility. For example, people may occupy schools 6–8 hr/day over a period of years, but for hospitals the occupancy may be continuous for 1 day or several months. These differences result in different pollutant exposures and effects.

PREVALENCE OF HEALTH CONDITIONS

People with health conditions that render them hypersusceptible to pollutant exposure are the most important high-risk groups. This is particularly the case when acute health impacts are being estimated. These are the first people affected by elevated pollutant concentrations, and they may be expected to have more obvious dose-response patterns than hypersusceptible populations estimated by facility or age. Unfortunately, direct estimates of prevalence (number of people with a given health condition) for local areas are not available, because of the high costs for surveys to develop them. Therefore, other methods must be used to obtain local prevalence estimates for the health conditions being measured.

At the national level prevalence estimates for various health conditions are available from the National Center for Health Statistics (NCHS) and are published in its "Vital and Health Statistics" series of reports. By applying the appropriate U.S. prevalence rate estimates to local population data the number of people in a specified area with a particular health condition can be estimated. However, the accuracy of the estimates will be determined by how closely the characteristics of the local population match the national sample.

The most simple application of this approach is to use the national crude prevalence rate for a given health condition as the local rate. This method has been the one most commonly used and, lacking other techniques, is probably the best available. It does not, however, take into account local differences in population characteristics (e.g., age or race), which have a significant influence on a condition's prevalence.

A technique called synthetic estimation has been developed and tested by the National Center for Health Statistics (NCHS) (4). This approach takes into account variations in local population characteristics. Local prevalence is estimated by dividing the population data into subgroups by characteristic (e.g., age, race, or sex) and applying specific prevalence rates (usually national level) to each of the subgroups. The subgroups are called demographic cells (α cells). The sum of the populations in the α cells is equal to the total local population. The total local prevalence of a health condition is the sum of the estimated prevalence in all of the demographic cells.

Using this technique two models for estimating the local prevalence of chronic bronchitis, emphysema, and asthma have been developed and tested (5). These diseases were selected because they are prevalent diseases in the United States today. Not only do chronic bronchitis, emphysema, and asthma have major impacts in disability and death, but also patients with one or more of these diseases are hypersusceptible to air pollutants affecting lung function (6).

The first model is simply a synthetic estimation. It uses local population data divided into cells by age, race, and sex and can therefore be used for any local area for which population data are available in that form. It is expressed as

$$\tilde{X}_{Ld} = \frac{10^5}{P_L} \sum_{\alpha=1}^{k} (p_{\alpha L} \bar{x}_{\alpha d}) \tag{3.1}$$

where

$\tilde{X}_{Ld}$ = the local synthetic estimate of prevalence rate per 100,000 population for disease d

$\bar{x}_{\alpha d}$ = the U.S. estimate of the proportion of the population in the αth cell with disease d

P_L = the total local population

d = the disease being estimated (chronic bronchitis, emphysema, or asthma)

$p_{\alpha L}$ = the local population in the αth cell.

The NCHS has developed U.S. prevalence rate estimates $\bar{x}_{\alpha d}$ for 1970 for each disease by age, race, and sex (7). They are given in Table 3.1.

The second model is designed to convert local death rate data into prevalence rate estimates. This is done by calculating estimates of local ratios of case fatality. These are ratios of the annual deaths from a disease to the number of cases of the disease. The case fatality ratios are then applied to local actual death rate data. The model is given as:

$$\tilde{X}'_{Ld} = \frac{\tilde{X}_{Ld}}{\tilde{Y}_{Ld}} (\bar{Y}_{Ld}) \tag{3.2}$$

Table 3.1 Estimated Proportion of U.S. Population with Chronic Bronchitis, Emphysema, and Asthma, by Age, Race, and Sex, 1970 ($\bar{x}_{\alpha d}$) (7)

Chronic Bronchitis		Under 17		17–44	45–64	65–over
W. male		0.0469		0.0175	0.0295	0.0493
W. female		0.0365		0.0308	0.0431	0.0375
All other		0.0227		0.0142	0.0235	0.0260[a]
Emphysema				Under 45		
W. male				0.0013	0.0238	0.0639
W. female				0.0009	0.0068	0.0124
All other				0.0001[a]	0.0043[a]	0.0026[a]
Asthma	Under 6		6–16	17–44		
W. male	0.0343		0.0373	0.0252	0.0281	0.0415
W. female	0.0211		0.0238	0.0274	0.0355	0.0306
All other	0.0364		0.0392	0.0252	0.0445	0.0429

[a] Figure does not meet NCHS standards of reliability or precision (>30% relative standard error).

where

$\tilde{X}'_{Ld}$ = death rate conversion estimate of local prevalence rate per 100,000 population for disease d

$\tilde{Y}_{Ld}$ = local synthetic estimate of deaths per 100,000 population for disease d.

$\bar{Y}_{Ld}$ = actual local death rate per 100,000 population for disease d.

The ratio of $\tilde{X}_{Ld}$ and $\tilde{Y}_{Ld}$ is a population-weighted ratio of cases to deaths, which converts an actual local disease death rate $\bar{Y}_{Ld}$ into a prevalence rate.

The synthetic death rate estimate $\tilde{Y}_{Ld}$ is of the same form as $\tilde{X}_{Ld}$ in (3.1). It is obtained by applying a cell-specific rate, $\bar{y}_{\alpha d}$ = the U.S. estimate of the proportion of the population in the αth cell dying annually from disease d. The U.S. death rates by age, race, and sex ($\bar{y}_{\alpha d}$) for 1970, obtained from the Census and Vital Statistics of the United States, are given in Table 3.2 (1,8). The α cells for $\bar{y}_{\alpha d}$ are identical to those for $\bar{x}_{\alpha d}$ given in Table 3.1, so the two sets may be used together in the model.

Table 3.2 U.S. Death Rates per 100,000 for Chronic Bronchitis, Emphysema, and Asthma, by Age, Race, and Sex, 1970 ($\bar{y}_{\alpha d} \cdot 10^5$) (1,8)

Chronic Bronchitis	Under 17		17–44	45–64	65–over
W. male	0.3509		0.2398	5.6570	36.5959
W. female	0.2456		0.1733	2.2030	8.4326
All other	0.6472		0.3357	3.5404	8.4718
Emphysema			**Under 45**		
W. male			0.2802	26.7338	168.9975
W. female			0.1762	6.3184	21.4513
All other			0.4392	10.5008	36.7689
Asthma	**Under 6**	**6–16**	**17–44**		
W. male	0.2441	0.1488	0.2705	1.5071	4.2246
W. female	0.1624	0.1662	0.5469	1.9837	3.6126
All other	0.7799	0.5812	2.0878	5.3949	5.5326

The second model was developed when it was ascertained that synthetic estimates of prevalence and mortality using age, race, and sex as determinants do not fully explain variations in actual local prevalence and mortality for these diseases. Equation (3.2) is expected to yield more accurate estimates than (3.1) for two reasons: (1) actual local mortality data is used to develop prevalence estimates; and (2) local population characteristics are taken into account when converting actual local death rates into predicted prevalence rates. In this model, local actual death rates averaged over a period of several years should be used to minimize the effects of random fluctuation over time in the local mortality data. If reliable mortality data are not available, the synthetic estimation model may be used.

Although the two prevalence rate estimation models yield biased estimates, they have predictive capabilities superior to that of crude rates applied to local populations and are useable with existing census, morbidity, and mortality data. The bias of the estimates is not affected by the size of the local population. Consequently, the models may be used for small areas or subareas to enumerate populations who are hypersusceptible to pollutant stress. The bias in the estimates is probably due to omission from the model of other disease determinants, for example, occupational exposures or smoking. This is true for both prevalence and death rate estimates and the ratios of case fatality calculated from them.

What determines the applicability of these models to any given location is the availability of local population and mortality data. Local population data by age, race, and sex is essential to the models, and the mortality data will enable better estimates to be made through use of the death rate conversion approach. If neither model can be applied, then crude U.S. rates are useful. Depending on the local population data, prevalence rates that are only specified by age or race may also be used. These will generate estimates that may be somewhat more accurate than those with the crude rates.

The synthetic estimation models discussed here were developed and tested only for chronic bronchitis, emphysema, and asthma. The same models can, however, be adapted to other health conditions for which U.S. prevalence rate estimates are available for specific demographic cells. The cell divisions are determined by those characteristics that have the greatest influence on a particular condition. Before applying this approach for other conditions, it must be tested using evaluative procedures similar to those used for these models (5). It should be determined if the models predict better than crude rates, how biased they are, and if their bias would be affected by the size or characteristics of the populations in the areas for which the prevalence of the condition will be estimated.

SAMPLE APPLICATION OF PREVALENCE ESTIMATION TECHNIQUES

The synthetic estimation models are demonstrated here by using both of them to estimate the prevalence rates and prevalence (number of people) for chronic bronchitis in 10 counties in a hypothetical geographical region. A third set of disease prevalence estimates was also calculated using the 1970 crude U.S. bronchitis prevalence rate of 3270 per 100,000 as the rate for each of the 10 counties.

The first step in the estimation procedure is to calculate the synthetic estimates of prevalence rates and death rates. This is done by multiplying the cell-specific rate for each cell by the population in that cell and summing the results for all cells in the total population. The rates used are

Table 3.3 Population and Synthetic Prevalence and Death Rate Estimates for Chronic Bronchitis by Age, Race, and Sex for County 1

	Under 17	17–44	45–64	Over 65
Population				
W. male	14341	11956	8614	2066
W. female	13783	13356	8437	2183
All other	295	386	343	90
Total = 76850				
Prevalence (number of persons)				
W. male	674	209	254	102
W. female	503	411	364	119
All other	7	5	8	2
Total = 2657 persons				
Prevalence Rate ($\tilde{X}_{L1}$) = 3458 per 100,000				
Death rate (per 100,000 total population)				
W. male	0.0655	0.0373	0.6341	0.9838
W. female	0.0440	0.0301	0.2419	0.3493
All other	0.0025	0.0017	0.0158	0.0099
Total ($\tilde{Y}_{L1}$) = 2.416 per 100,000				

the proportions of prevalence $\bar{x}_{\alpha d}$ and deaths $\bar{y}_{\alpha d}$ for chronic bronchitis, given in Tables 3.1 and 3.2 respectively. An example of this procedure for county 1 is demonstrated in Table 3.3 which gives the cell-specific populations and the prevalence and death rates resulting from the calculations.

The development of the synthetic estimate and death rate conversion estimate for county 1 are shown in Table 3.4. The synthetic estimates are the prevalence and prevalence rate calculated and presented in Table 3.3. For the death rate conversion estimate, the prevalence and death rate estimates are used to calculate the ratio of cases to deaths, which is then multiplied by the actual local bronchitis death rate (in this case, a three-year average rate) to yield an estimated prevalence rate.

Results of these calculations performed for each of the 10 hypothetical counties are presented in Table 3.5, along with the estimated prevalence calculated using the crude U.S. bronchitis prevalence rate. Different patterns of disease prevalence (both rates and numbers of people) are obtained from each method. As shown in Table 3.5, the prevalence rates for the 10 counties for the death rate conversion estimates range from

Table 3.4 Synthetic and Death Rate Conversion Estimates of Chronic Bronchitis Prevalence in County 1

	Intermediate Results	Prevalence Rate per 100,000	Prevalence (no. of people)
Synthetic estimation		3458	2657
Death rate conversion			
$\tilde{X}_{L1}$ (per 100,000)	3458		
$\tilde{Y}_{L1}$ (per 100,000)	2.416		
Ratio of cases to deaths	1431		
Actual bronchitis death rate per 100,000 ($\bar{Y}_{L1}$)	1.910		
Prevalence estimates		2734	2101

Table 3.5 Prevalence and Prevalence Rate Estimates for Chronic Bronchitis by Three Estimation Methods

	Synthetic Estimates		Death Rate Conversion		Crude Estimate
County	Prevalence Rate $\tilde{X}_{L1}$	Prevalence (number of people)	Prevalence Rate $\tilde{X}'_{L1}$	Prevalence (number of people)	Prevalence (number of people)
1	3458	2,657	2743	2,101	2,513
2	3443	3,125	2233	2,027	2,968
3	3215	3,050	1919	1,821	3,102
4	3408	3,702	2291	2,489	3,552
5	3450	4,125	1881	2,249	3,910
6	3469	3,870	3968	4,427	3,648
7	3411	5,503	4516	7,286	5,276
8	3334	8,222	3475	8,570	8,065
9	3376	8,474	2929	7,352	8,208
10	3402	16,734	2668	13,123	16,085
Total prevalence		59,462		51,445	57,327
Average prevalence rate (per 100,000)		3,391		2,935	3,270

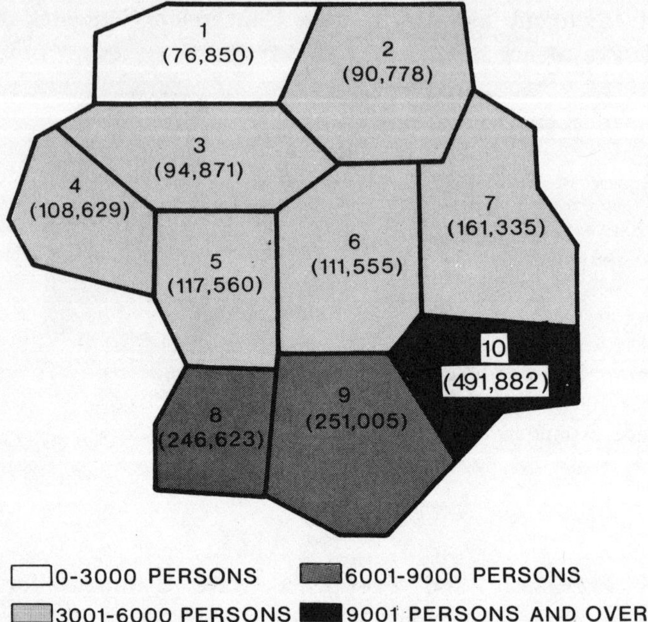

Figure 3.1. Distribution of county chronic bronchitis prevalence estimates calculated by use of the synthetic estimation method. (County population given in parentheses)

1881 to 4516/100,000. In contrast to this rather wide distribution, all 10 counties have the same crude rate estimate (which is 3270/100,000), and there is a narrow range in estimates (from 3215 to 3469/100,000) for the synthetic estimates of prevalence rates.

A wider distribution for prevalence values is observed, reflecting the wide range of populations in the 10 counties (76,850 to 491,882 total population) from which they are calculated. The three distributions of synthetic estimates, death rate conversion estimates, and crude estimates of prevalence are highlighted in Figures 3.1 through 3.3. These figures and Table 3.5 show that the death rate conversion estimates are the most conservative estimates and that the synthetic estimation yields the highest values. The total prevalence rate estimates for the entire region, however, are quite similar for the three methods, ranging from 2935 to 3391 per 100,000 total population.

Because the death rate conversion method is based on actual mortality data, which is converted to prevalence rate estimates by use of population-weighted ratios of cases to death, this method is expected to

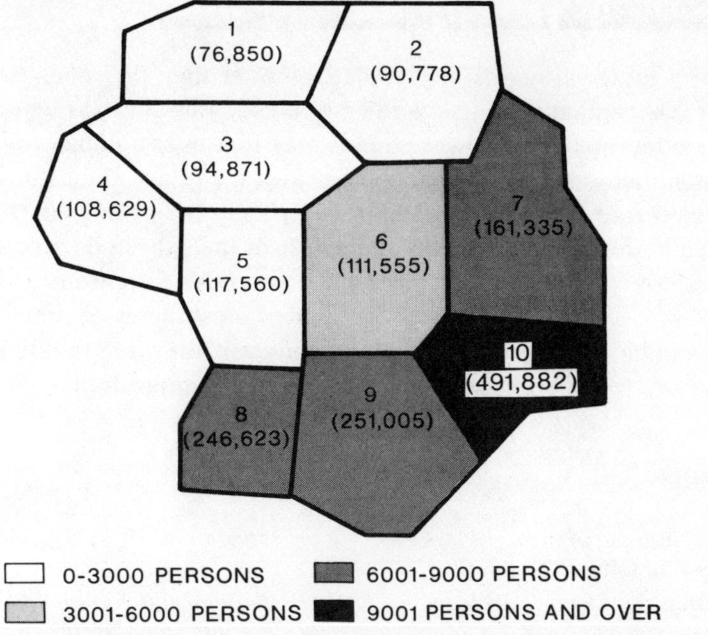

Figure 3.2. Distribution of county chronic bronchitis prevalence estimates calculated by use of the death rate conversion method. (County population given in parentheses)

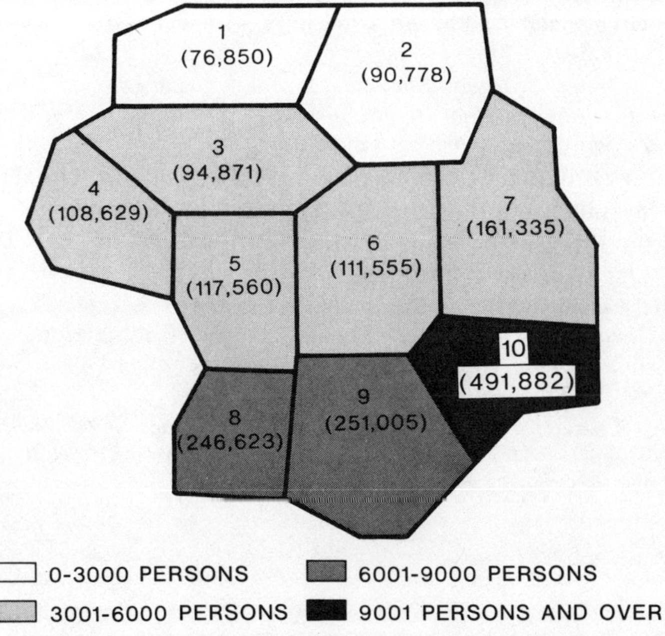

Figure 3.3. Distribution of county chronic bronchitis prevalence estimates calculated by use of the U.S. crude prevalence rate estimate. (County population given in parentheses)

quantify local variations in prevalence better than the other two procedures. The similarity of its overall prevalence rate for the region to those of the other methods, however, indicates that over a number of samples all three methods should yield similar average rates. The estimates from the death rate conversion method will usually be lower than those from the synthetic estimation method, because of the expected tendency of the latter to overestimate prevalence and death rates for chronic obstructive lung disease. In this example, the synthetic estimates of prevalence are quite similar to the crude estimates. However, they do provide improved sensitivity to differences in local population composition.

REFERENCES

1. U.S. Bureau of the Census. *Census of the Population: 1970*. U.S. Government Printing Office, Washington, DC, 1973.
2. Farley, D. O. and Wadden, R. A. *An Environmental Health Evaluation of Highway Networks—A Methodological Development*. Northeastern Illinois Planning Commission, Chicago. National Technical Information Service No. PB242-378/AS, 1974.
3. Wadden, R. A., Farley, D. O., and Carnow, B. W. Transportation emissions and environmental health: An evaluatory planning methodology. *Environ. Plann. A*, **8**:3–21, 1976.
4. National Center for Health Statistics. *Synthetic State Estimates of Disability: Derived from the National Health Survey*. PHS Pub. No. 1759, U.S. Government Printing Office, Washington, DC, 1968.
5. Farley, D. O., Wadden, R. A., and Levy, P. S. Estimation of local prevalence of chronic obstructive lung disease. Submitted for publication.
6. American Lung Association. *Chronic Obstructive Pulmonary Disease, A Manual for Physicians*. New York, 1973.
7. National Center for Health Statistics. *Prevalence of Selected Chronic Respiratory Conditions, United States, 1970*. Vital and Health Statistics, PHS Pub. No. 1000-Series 10, No. 84. U.S. Government Printing Office, Washington, DC, Sept. 1973.
8. National Center for Health Statistics. *Vital Statistics of the United States: 1970. Volume II—Mortality*. U.S. DHEW Pub. No. (HRA) 75-1101, Rockville, MD, 1974.

QUANTITATING THE EFFECTS OF ENVIRONMENTAL STRESS

4

ALTERATIONS IN DISEASE RATES

Anneke de Werk Neal

There are several approaches to obtaining quantitative information on relationships between exposure to pollutants and human health effects. Toxicologic studies with animals permit the careful control of the most important variables (covariates), the utilization of a wide range of exposures, and the examination of body tissues. However, there are difficulties in extrapolating animal data to humans. Clinical or laboratory studies of human patients or volunteers may permit some control of covariates, but a wide range of exposure levels and times is not easily evaluated. Epidemiologic studies investigate the health effects of complex long-term and short-term pollutant exposure on susceptible human groups. Examination of variations in disease or mortality rates between population groups exposed to different levels of a particular pollutant is used to quantitatively determine the extent to which environmental pollutants affect human health. Epidemiologic studies, however, must deal with a host of interacting covariates and are restricted to a limited range of exposures. The assessment of adverse health effects from pollutant exposure is most effectively accomplished by using all the research approaches presented above. This discussion, however, focuses on the epidemiologic approach. Chapters 5 and 6 cover body burden and physiological changes that are detected and measured by toxicologic and clinical studies.

Epidemiology is the study of disease occurrence in human population groups. Epidemiologic investigations of pollution health effects attempt to determine the associations between levels of specific pollutant exposures and the rate of mortality or disease, or the occurrence of physiologic changes in body functions, within population groups.

Epidemiologic studies are carried out in a natural environment. These investigations involve the collection of extensive information on observed exposure levels and disease frequency. The population groups examined may be "natural," such as communities, cities, or nations, the occupationally exposed, or people hypersusceptible to certain diseases. Observational studies fall into two major types, retrospective and prospective. In a retrospective study people diagnosed as having a disease (cases) and people without the disease (controls) are compared with respect to past exposure to pollutants. A major problem with this method of study is that information on past pollution levels may be incomplete or inaccurate. In prospective studies populations (cohorts) free of the disease of interest are subdivided according to different pollutant exposure levels and followed, over time, for development of disease. A third design, the historical prospective or longitudinal study, is actually prospective in approach. It utilizes a previously assembled cohort, such as all employees of a given industry, classifies individuals in the cohort according to past exposure, and observes their subsequent morbidity or mortality for a period of time. However, such a study also relies upon past pollutant exposure data. Most of the epidemiologic studies presented in this chapter are cohort studies of the longitudinal type. This is primarily because information on pollution exposure and associated disease, in the detail required for applying the retrospective approach, has generally not been available in the past.

In epidemiologic studies an association between pollutant exposure and an adverse health effect is most likely to be causal if it is consistent with overall biological knowledge; if it can be demonstrated by more than one research approach; if it is consistently observed by different investigators and in different places; and if increased exposure levels are accompanied by increased frequency of the disorder. The latter is commonly referred to as a dose-response or exposure-effect relationship. The purpose of many environmental epidemiologic studies is to define a dose-response relationship for variables suspected or known to be causally associated. Not only does a dose-response effect strengthen a causal association, but it also can be used to estimate the expected amount of disease and mortality associated with measured concentrations of individual, or groups of, pollutants.

The primary purpose of this discussion is to present several known environmental dose-response relationships that relate alterations in disease rates and mortality rates to pollution levels. An attempt has been made to include various hypersusceptible groups. Before setting forth any specific relationships several important imperfections in epidemiologic studies, and consequent limitations of the resulting data, should be noted:

1. Accurate estimation of human exposure based on environmental monitoring data can be difficult because of the varied spatial and temporal activities of those being studied.
2. An inadequate number of sampling sites, inaccurate methods of measurement, and failure to consider meteorological conditions can lead to error in estimation of pollutant exposure.
3. The health effects studies on which dose-response relationships are based are limited by shortcomings of vital records and by error in measurement of disease.
4. In comparing disease or death rates of people it is often difficult, and in some cases impossible, to control and evaluate disease-related factors such as socioeconomic status; smoking habits; occupational exposure to pollutants; the heterogeneous nature of the health of a diverse population; previous exposure to pollutants; medical history; nutritional status; and different climatic conditions.
5. Long latency periods between exposure and disease can obscure relationships between the two.
6. The different effects of infrequent short-term peak exposures, long-term exposures, and frequent short-term exposures are difficult to take into account.
7. The relationships between exposure and disease are further complicated by the possibility of: (*a*) a single environmental agent contributing to a number of different disorders and (*b*) a single disorder resulting from a combination of agents.

Unfortunately, past epidemiologic studies have not been able to control for many of the significant factors cited above. However, as more sophisticated investigative and data analysis techniques are developed, better assessment of pollution-health effects may become available. In applying dose-response relationships based on one population group to another, the difference in important characteristics between the two groups should be minimized. It is necessary to give careful consideration to whom the relationships apply. Despite these limitations such a dose-response approach does provide a means for preliminary quantitation of environmental stress. The pollutants discussed in this chapter are sulfur dioxide (SO_2), suspended sulfates, total suspended particulates (TSP), lead (Pb), and coal tar pitch volatiles (CTPV).

SULFUR DIOXIDE: ACUTE RESPIRATORY ILLNESS IN CHILDREN

Sulfur dioxide is known to be a respiratory irritant. The irritant effect probably results from the conversion of SO_2 to sulfurous acid in the presence of water in the lung. When SO_2 is experienced in association with particulates, it may be absorbed onto the surfaces of respirable aerosols and carried into the lower respiratory tract. There the droplets may be transformed into more highly irritant substances such as sulfuric acid and metallic sulfates. It is believed that all atmospheric SO_2 is eventually oxidized to sulfates either in the gas phase or after absorption by plants or absorption onto surfaces (1).

Acute respiratory illness is an important multibillion dollar public health problem and is identified as the leading cause of acute morbidity in the United States (2). Children experience a much higher rate of incidence of acute respiratory disease than the population at large and hence have been the focus of a number of environmental epidemiologic studies. Two such evaluations, prospective surveys in New York (3) and Chicago (2) of acute respiratory disease conducted through the Environmental Protection Agency's (EPA) CHESS program, provide the basis for Figure 4.1. These studies were combined because the data were collected, analyzed, and presented in a similar manner; because the subjects were comparable in socioeconomic and other factors; and because the mix of pollutants in the two cities was not too different. The attack rates of upper and lower respiratory disease in children were obtained by telephone interviews with the mothers. The Chicago data (over 600 children) were collected over a period of 46 weeks (1969–1970). The New York study (300 children) lasted 30 weeks (1970–1971), and both study periods included an influenza season. The rates in Figure 4.1 have been adjusted to

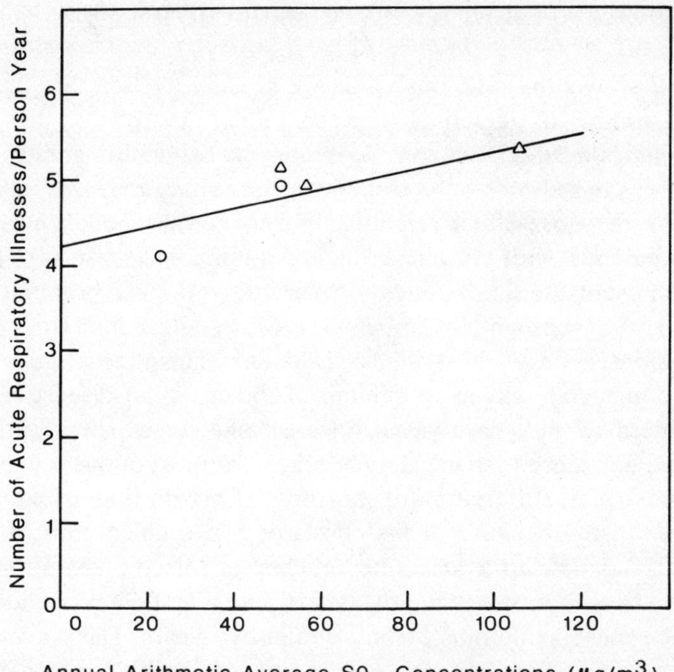

Figure 4.1. Frequency of acute respiratory disease in children under 5 years versus annual SO_2 concentration [from (2, 3)]. △ Chicago Study; ○ New York Study.

extend over a period of one year. Because the studies ran during seasons with the highest illness rates, extrapolation of these data to one year may be a little high. All children in both studies resided within 1.5 miles of an air monitoring station. The children in Chicago were divided into three residential pollution exposure categories as measured by air monitoring stations during 1969–1970. The annual arithmetic average SO_2 concentration in the "intermediate" exposure area was 57 $\mu g/m^3$ (with 111 μg TSP/m^3); in the "high" area it was 51 $\mu g/m^3$ (with 126 μg TSP/m^3), and in the "highest" it was 106 $\mu g/m^3$ (with 151 μg TSP/m^3). The New York children resided in a "low" pollution area where the annual average SO_2 concentration was 23 $\mu g/m^3$ and annual average TSP level was 34 $\mu g/m^3$, or they resided in an "intermediate" area with annual averages of 51 μg SO_2/m^3 and 63–86 μg TSP/m^3.

SULFUR DIOXIDE: CHEST ILLNESS IN BRONCHITICS

Figure 4.2 shows the relationship between daily average SO_2 levels and expected number of person-days of chest illness per person-day of exposure for males aged 55 and over with chronic bronchitis grades 3 and 4. This figure is based on results from a Chicago study that was designed to investigate the dose-effect relationship between air pollution and morbidity in patients with chronic bronchopulmonary disease (4). The data points represent the illness days of over 100 volunteer bronchitics from October 1, 1967 through November 30, 1967, as determined from patients' daily responses on a chest illness calendar. The illness calendar was organized in such a way as to minimize subjectivity of disease reporting. Chest illness or sick day was defined as one on which a patient was bothered much more than usual by his chest for most of the day, had more cough than usual, suffered more shortness of breath than usual, was less active than usual because of his chest, or had a chest cold. A grade 3 bronchitic was defined as one who coughed or raised phlegm throughout the day and year for more than two years, and a grade 4 bronchitic had to experience these symptoms for more than five years. Daily average SO_2 concentrations in each patient's square mile of employment or residence were estimated, based on SO_2 measurements made at eight city-wide

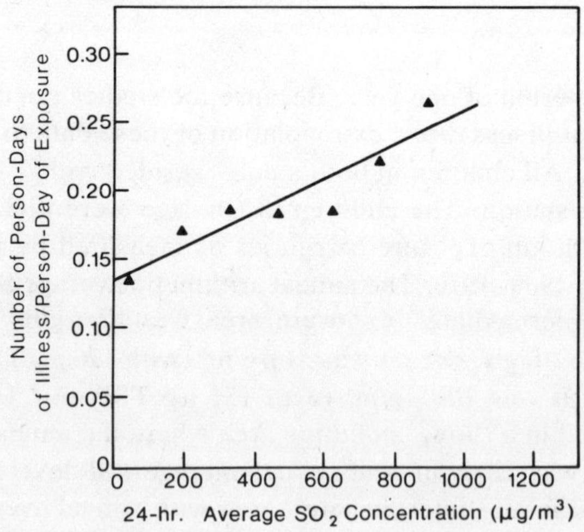

Figure 4.2. Frequency of illness days in males over 55 years with grade 3 and 4 bronchitis versus daily SO_2 concentrations [data from (4)].

continuous monitoring stations. Figure 4.2 was derived by dividing the number of person-days of chest illness occurring one day after exposure to a particular pollution concentration by the number of person-days of exposure at that level. The selection of the fall study period (as opposed to winter) avoided the problem of severe low temperatures complicating health effects, and the problem of bronchitics experiencing less outdoor exposure during the winter. In applying these data to a study group for an environmental impact evaluation, it would be desirable to define a group in the same age bracket, with similar degrees of bronchitis, and residing in similar urban settings.

SULFUR DIOXIDE: MORTALITY

Figure 4.3 is a graph showing a stepwise dose-response relationship between mortality and SO_2 concentrations. This figure represents the results of a study (5) that evaluated daily variations in the death rate for the New York metropolitan area for 1962–1966 in relation to the air quality data as measured at one monitoring station. The application of air quality data from one station to an entire metropolitan region renders this relationship as rather imprecise, even though the investigators adjusted the death rates for seasonal cycles, temperature fluctuations, and other confounding variables. Figure 4.3 indicates that on days when SO_2 levels were above 500 $\mu g/m^3$ mortality was approximately 2% greater than

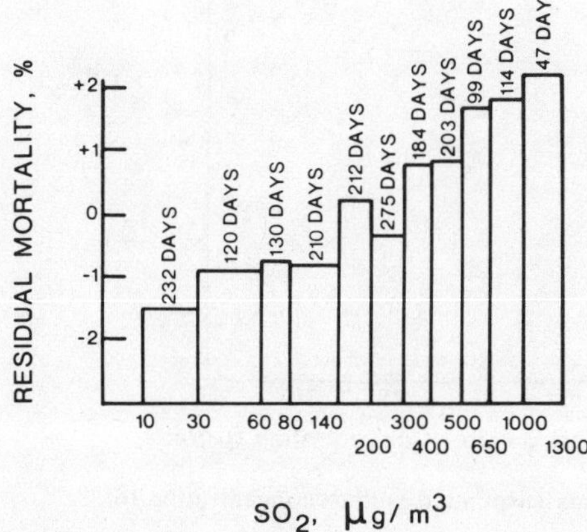

Figure 4.3. Means of residual mortality by SO_2 levels, 1962–1966 (1826 Days) [from (5)].

expected. For days when SO_2 concentrations were below 30 $\mu g/m^3$ mortality was 1.5% less than expected.

SUSPENDED SULFATES: ASTHMATICS

Figure 4.4 presents temperature-specific dose-response relationships for suspended sulfate levels and resultant asthma attack rates in New York (6). A panel of 148 asthmatics recorded asthma attacks in a daily diary from October 1970 through May 1971. All subjects lived within 1.5 miles of a monitoring station and were divided among three communities of differing air quality. Average daily suspended sulfate concentrations were obtained by analyzing total suspended particulates for the sulfate fraction using a turbidimetric method. The resultant dose-response function plotted in Figure 4.4 predicts that a suspended sulfate exposure of 35 $\mu g/m^3$ would be associated with a 4% increase in asthma attacks on cooler days (30°F < minimum temperature, t_{min} < 50°F) and 57% increase on warmer days (t_{min} > 50°F). When using these relationships, it should be recog-

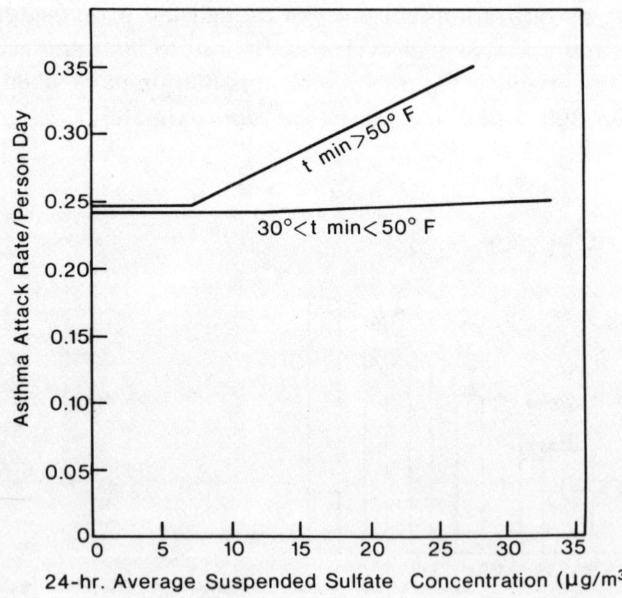

Figure 4.4. Asthma attack rate versus suspended sulfate concentration (6).

nized that the study did not include the effect of plant allergens nor the potential effect of other pollutants.

TOTAL SUSPENDED PARTICULATES: MORTALITY FROM CHRONIC RESPIRATORY DISEASE

The toxicological action of particulate matter may occur in several ways: (1) the particles may be intrinsically toxic; (2) they may interfere with clearance mechanisms in the respiratory tract; and (3) the particles may interact with, or act as a carrier of, toxic material. Figure 4.5 relates the average annual death rate from chronic respiratory disease to particulate pollution levels measured in the Buffalo area (7). A strong correlation was found between chronic respiratory disease mortality in white males 50–69 years old and suspended particulate levels, regardless of the economic level of the deceased. Total suspended particulate concentrations were measured at 21 air sampling stations in and around Buffalo from July 1961 until June 1963. These data resulted in the designation of four particulate exposure areas: the low-exposure area had a 2-year geometric mean of 80 μg TSP/m^3; level 2, 80–100 μg/m^3; level 3, 100–135 μg/m^3; and level 4 was > 135 μg/m^3. Mortality data for the study area were obtained for the period 1959–1961 using the 1960 census as the population basis. Figure 4.5

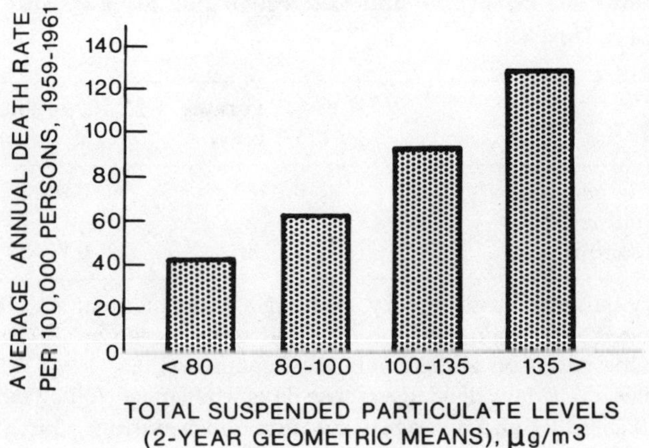

Figure 4.5. Average annual death rate from chronic respiratory disease for white males (Age 50–69) versus total particulate matter concentrations (7).

indicates that the death rate from chronic respiratory disease was 44 per 100,000 persons in the lowest pollution area, almost 40% higher for persons in the next most polluted area, and approximately three times as high for persons at the highest pollution level.

In this study no consideration was given to occupation. Other limitations of the analysis included the inability to obtain information on the deceased's smoking habits and the uncertainty that the pollution levels are representative of exposure at the time the chronic disease conditions were developing.

GRAIN DUST (SUSPENDED PARTICULATES): ASTHMA INCIDENCE

A University of Minnesota study investigated the relationship between air pollution generated by grain handling and processing facilities and allergic diseases (8). Grain sensitive students were found to experience a statistically significantly higher incidence of bronchial asthma attacks on days when the grain air pollution was high (when mean soiling index was greater than 0.25 Coefficient of Haze (COH)) and the average wind direction was from a large grain processing plant to student housing areas, than on all other days. These results are shown in Table 4.1. Although the data

Table 4.1 Asthma Incidence among Students during Conditions Favorable and Less Favorable for Exposure to Grain Dust (8)

Groups[a]	Less Favorable (157 days)	Favorable[b] (68 days)
Grain sensitive	0.0320	0.0520[c]
Grain negative (control)	0.0280	0.0340[d]

[a] 126 students with history of allergic bronchial asthma were divided into grain positive (51) and grain negative (75) subgroups based on allergic skin test reactions.
[b] Favorable days defined as those days when mean soiling index > 0.25 COH and average wind direction was from source to student residences.
[c] Standard error of the difference = ± 0.0062, $p < 0.001$.
[d] Not significant.

are limited, they do provide a basis for a dose-response evaluation that combines pollution concentrations and wind direction.

LEAD: BLOOD LEAD LEVELS IN CHILDREN

The results of an Idaho lead study (9) are an example of the relationship that may exist between environmental exposure and subclinical physiologic changes within a specific population group. Children were the focal subjects of this study because of the high susceptibility of their nervous systems to the effects of Pb.

Five concentric study areas were defined at various distances (1 to 20 miles) from a primary lead smelter in northern Idaho. In addition two control areas were designated; one a rural logging town 45 miles northwest of the smelter and the other a side valley southwest of the smelter. A survey of blood levels among 1074 children, aged 1–9 years, residing in the seven study areas was conducted in August of 1974. Information on age, sex, length of residence at current and previous address, pica history, parents' occupation and education level, and physical conditions of the home environment were obtained for each child. An extensive air monitoring system provided information for a model used to estimate the Pb exposure for the subject children. Nine high-volume samplers were run for 24-hr periods every other day to determine an annual ambient air Pb concentration in each of the seven study areas for August 1973 to August 1974. For each child's home samples of surface soil, inside and outside home dust and paint, and grass and garden vegetables were tested for Pb level. Using multiple regression analysis, ambient air Pb, soil Pb, age of child, cleanliness of home, and parent occupation (measured as social status) were found to significantly ($p < 0.0001$) influence blood Pb levels. Ambient air Pb was found to be the most strongly related variable, and Table 4.2 presents the data for the air-Pb-blood-Pb relationship. Soil Pb was the second most significant variable, and the soil-Pb-blood-Pb data are shown in Table 4.3.

COAL TAR PITCH VOLATILES: LUNG CANCER MORTALITY AMONG COKE OVEN WORKERS

Epidemiologic studies of occupational groups in their work setting have been important in establishing dose-response relationships for many pol-

Table 4.2 Mean Blood Pb Levels in Children Related to Ambient Air Pb Exposure (9)

Mean Annual Ambient Air Pb Concentration[a] ($\mu g/m^3$)	Geometric Mean Blood Pb Level[b] (μg/100 ml)
0.5	21.0
0.55	30.3
0.6	27.6
3.0	32.3
7.0	33.8
14.4	47.4
16.8	65.6

[a] For period August 1973 to August 1974.
[b] Measured in 1074 children aged 1–9 years, August 1974.

lutants. Occupational studies generally offer a better-defined cohort, a wider range of pollutant exposures, and higher levels of exposure than community studies. However, it is difficult to apply occupational dose-response relationships to environmental evaluations because community exposures are generally 24 hr/day compared to 8 hr/day; community exposures begin at birth rather than age of employment; and the occupationally exposed may not include as many hypersusceptible individuals as the general population. However, in the absence of environmental studies, work-related exposure analyses may be useful in evaluating pollutant

Table 4.3 Mean Blood Pb Levels in Children Related to Soil Pb Content (9)

Mean Pb Content of Surface Soils[a] (ppm)	Geometric Mean Blood Pb Level[b] (μg/100 ml)
300	21.0
600	30.3
1250	33.8
1375	32.3
2250	27.6
3300	47.4
7700	65.6

[a] Measured in 1974.
[b] Measured in 1074 children aged 1–9 years, August 1974.

health effects. The following study of coke oven workers is included as an example of an occupational epidemiologic study.

Coal tar pitch volatiles (CTPV) represent the gaseous discharge of coke ovens used in the steel industry. Benzo(a)pyrene, a known animal carcinogen, is a major component of CTPV. Lloyd analyzed the lung cancer mortality of coke oven workers and found excess risk of lung cancer for this occupation (10). Data were obtained on 4661 coke oven workers (1979 white, 2682 nonwhite) from 12 steel plants in the United States for the years 1951–1966. Information on specific jobs held by each man, length of time in each job, race, age, and date and cause of death (when applicable) was compiled. CTPV levels were measured for specific job sites at 10 coke oven installations. A considerable difference in exposure was noted for the various job locations.

Using these data, an epidemiologic study has been carried out on the relationship between cumulative exposure to CTPV and lung cancer mortality (11). Using individual work histories (the length of time in different work areas and the level of exposure in those areas) an index of cumulative exposure was calculated for each worker. For example, a worker exposed to 0.56 mg/m^3 for 30 years would accumulate approximately 200 mg/m^3-months of CTPV. Lung cancer mortality rates observed during 1951–1966 were tabulated for four CTPV exposure intervals with age adjustment for the total rates and with an age-specific breakdown. A strong positive relationship between level of CTPV exposure and lung cancer mortality was observed for nonwhites (Table 4.4). This dose-response relationship is shown in Figure 4.6. It should be mentioned that lung cancer has a 15 to 25-year latent period. The study population was observed for only 14 years, so the health effects estimates should be considered conservative. Also, no smoking data were available. However, it has been argued that lung cancer mortality rates among top-side coke oven workers exceed expected levels even if all coke oven workers were heavy smokers (11).

SUMMARY

The foregoing examples represent some of the more recent and better-defined dose-response relationships based on epidemiologic evaluations. Although complicated and imprecise, epidemiologic studies do measure the ultimate effect of pollution on populations, rather than the theoretical effect extrapolated from animal or laboratory investigations. The limita-

Table 4.4 Age-Adjusted and Age-Specific Lung Cancer Mortality Rates[a] for White and Nonwhite Coke Oven Workers by Cumulative CTPV Exposure and Age at Entry to Study (11)

Age at Entry to Study (years)	Rate/1000									
			Cumulative CTPV exposure (mg/m³-months)							
	No Exposure[b]		≤ 199		200–499		500–699		700+	
	White	Non-white	White	Non-white	White	Non-white	White	Non-white	White[d]	Non-white
<35	0.8	1.1	0	1.7	2.7	9.6	0	7.9	0	45.5
35–44	5.7	3.4	13.9	0	7.8	10.0	36.4	20.0	0	42.1
45–54	18.2	19.6	66.7	18.5	28.3	19.9	0	46.3	0	51.6
>54	25.8	7.9	0	0	29.4	29.0	50.0	105.3	0	169.5
Total[c]	7.0	5.5	15.4	4.0	10.5	12.9	13.5	24.9	—	54.6

[a] Based on mortality observed during 1951–1966.
[b] Men who never worked at or on coke ovens before or after entry into study.
[c] Age-adjusted rate based on the age distribution of nonwhite coke oven workers.
[d] Only 62 workers were in this exposure category.

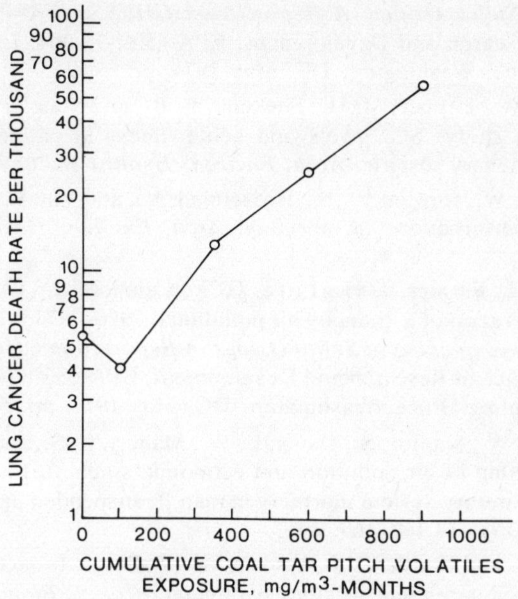

Figure 4.6. Age-adjusted lung cancer death rates among nonwhite coke oven workers by cumulative coal tar pitch volatile exposure, 1951–1966 (11).

tions of these studies should be recognized when dose-response relationships are applied. However, at the minimum, they do provide an important means for preliminary quantitation of human health effects of pollutant exposure.

REFERENCES

1. Rall, D. P. Review of the health effects of sulfur oxides. *Environ. Health Perspect.* **8**:98–121, 1974.
2. Finklea, J. F., French, J. G., Lowrimore, G. R., Goldberg, J., Shy, C. M., and Nelson, W. C. Prospective surveys of acute respiratory disease in volunteer families: Chicago nursery school study 1969–1970. In *Health Consequences of Sulfur Oxides: A Report from CHESS, 1970–1971*. U.S. EPA Office of Research and Development, EPA-650/1-74-004. U.S. Government Printing Office, Washington, DC, May 1974, pp. 4-37–4-55.
3. Love, J. G., Cohen, A. A., Finklea, J. F., French, J. G., Lowrimore, G. R., Nelson, W. C., and Ramsey, P. B. Prospective surveys of acute respiratory disease in volunteer families: 1970–1971 New York studies. In *Health Conse-*

quences of Sulfur Oxides: A Report from CHESS, 1970–1971. U.S. EPA Office of Research and Development, EPA-650/1-74-004. U.S. Government Printing Office, Washington, DC, May 1974, pp. 5-49–5-69.

4. Carnow, B. W., Lepper, M. H., Shekelle, R. B., and Stamler, J. The Chicago air pollution study: SO_2 levels and acute illness in patients with chronic bronchopulmonary disease. *Arch. Environ. Health*. **18**:768–776, 1969.
5. Buechley, R. W., Riggan, W. B., Hasselblad, V., and Van Bruggen, J. B. SO_2 levels and perturbations in mortality. *Arch. Environ. Health*. **27**:134–137, 1973.
6. Finklea, J. F., Farmer, J. H., Love, G. J., Calafiore, D. C., and Sovocool, G. W. Aggravation of asthma by air pollutants: 1970–1971 New York studies. In *Health Consequences of Sulfur Oxides: A Report from CHESS, 1970–1971*. U.S. EPA Ofice of Research and Development, EPA-650/1-74-004. U.S. Government Printing Office, Washington, DC, May 1974, pp. 5-71–5-84.
7. Winkelstein, W., Kantor, S., Davis, E. W., Maneri, C. S., and Mosher, W. E. The relationship of air pollution and economic status to total mortality and selected respiratory system mortality in man. I. suspended particulates. *Arch. Environ. Health*. **14**:162–169, 1967.
8. Paulus, H. J. and Smith, T. J. Association of allergic bronchial asthma with certain air pollutants and weather parameters. *Int. J. Biometeorol.* **11**:119–127, 1967.
9. Yankel, A. J., von Lindern, I. H., and Walter, S. D. The Silver Valley lead study: Lead levels and environmental exposure. *J. Air Pollut. Control Assoc.* **27**:763–767, 1977.
10. Lloyd, J. W. Long-term mortality study of steelworkers, V. Respiratory cancer in coke plant workers. *J. Occup. Med.* **13**:53–68, 1971.
11. Mazumdar, S., Redmond, C., Sollecito, W., and Sussman, N. An epidemiological study of exposure to coal tar pitch volatiles among coke oven workers. *J. Air Pollut. Control Assoc.* **25**:382–389, 1975.

5

BODY BURDEN

Alvin L. Miller

Body burden is the amount of element or compound in the body at any time, usually expressed in units of weight, for example, micrograms (or for radioactive material, microcuries). The total body burden at any time is due to the sum of exposures from many sources such as hobbies, food, dishes, and the ambient and occupational environment. Total body burden is the sum of the burdens for all the individual organs, one or more of which may be considered as critical organs.

A critical body organ is that organ of the body which when damaged by a pollutant results in the greatest damage to the body. It is readily apparent that many factors must be considered in determining which affected organ will cause the body to suffer the greatest damage. The criteria of prime importance in determining which organ is critical are (1):

1. The organ that accumulates the greatest concentration of the pollutant.
2. The essentialness or indispensability of the organ to the well-being of the entire body.
3. The organ damaged by the route of entry of the material into the body.
4. The sensitivity of the organs, that is, the organ damaged by the lowest dose.

Table 5.1 Critical Organs and Some Related Toxic Agents

Organ Systems	Toxic Agents
Brain	Methyl mercury; organic lead; carbon monoxide; mercury; manganese
Nasopharyngeal	Cadmium; arsenic; nickel; chromium
Lungs	Manganese; magnesium; beryllium; zinc; asbestos; sulfur oxides; ammonia; cadmium; ozone; nitrogen oxides; peroxyacetyl nitrate; nickel carbonate; hydrogen sulfide
Liver	Selenium; chlorinated hydrocarbons
Kidney	Mercury; cadmium; lead
Bone	Flouride; lead; strontium; radium; plutonium
Skin	Arsenic; beryllium; nickel; chromium
Fat	Chlorinated hydrocarbons (e.g., DDT)
Gastro-intestinal	Zinc; lead; arsenic; fluoride; vanadium
Thyroid	Cobalt; iodine
Heart	Carbon monoxide

Table 5.1 gives some examples of toxic agents and their respective critical organs.

Two prime factors that affect body organ burden are the environment to which the individual is exposed and the characteristics of the individual. The two principal components in the body burden relationship due to exposure in the environment are uptake and elimination. Uptake can be defined:

$$\text{uptake} = (\text{intake})\ (\text{fraction retained or deposited}) \qquad (5.1)$$

Intake, the amount inhaled or ingested per unit of time, for example, micrograms per day, is directly related to the concentrations in air, water, and food. Therefore these concentrations are some of the principal factors of concern. Body burden estimates are usually based on "reference man." Because of anatomical and physiological differences among individuals, mean values for such things as body weight, blood composition, and volume are used for calculations. For example, reference man weighs 70 kg and has a liver weight of 1.8 kg. He inhales 20 m^3 of air per day and ingests 2.2 liters of water per day (2). The amount of pollutant inhaled or ingested may be estimated in the following manner:

$$
\begin{aligned}
\text{total ingested} &= \text{mass from water} + \text{mass from food} && (5.2)\\
&= \text{(volume of water ingested) (concentration in water)}\\
&\quad + \text{(mass of food) (concentration in food)}\\
\text{total inhaled} &= \text{mass from air} && (5.3)\\
&= \text{(volume inhaled) (air concentration)}\\
\text{total intake} &= \text{total ingested} + \text{total inhaled} && (5.4)
\end{aligned}
$$

One may inhale and/or ingest the same material from many sources. Each contributes to the total body burden. In addition, the nature of the material must be considered. That is, is it in a gas or particulate form? What is its chemical structure and its solubility in body fluids? If it is in particulate form, the particle size distribution must be considered in determining the amount of pollutant that can penetrate into the various regions of the lung (3).

Even when the environmental exposure is the same, two individuals may have greatly different body burdens. This difference may be attributed in large part to differences in age and sex of the individuals, level of physical activity, presence of respiratory disease, difference in breathing pattern, and nutrition.

SINGLE COMPARTMENT MODELS

When an element is ingested or inhaled it may be deposited in one or more organs. If more than one organ is involved this would represent more than one compartment. Generally, then, a compartment may be considered to be an organ or organ system. There are two rather simplified models for estimating body burdens. These have been used particularly by the International Commission on Radiation Protection (ICRP) (1,4,5). The models are: (1) continuous exposure to a constant concentration of a specific material with exponential elimination from a single compartment; and (2) single intake of a specific material over a short period of time (hours) with exponential elimination from a single compartment.

Definition of Terms

m = mass of organ

C = mass ratio in organ, mass of pollutant per unit mass of organ

mC = body or organ burden, mass of pollutant
f_a = fraction of pollutant inhaled that reaches the organ of reference
f_w = fraction of pollutant ingested that reaches the organ of reference
I = average mass of pollutant inhaled or ingested per day
T_b = biological half-life, time required for half of material to be eliminated from organ or body
T_e = Effective half-life for radioactive materials
k = $0.693/T_b$, fraction eliminated per unit of time

Continuous Exposure

The model for continuous exposure (for ingestion only) at constant concentration with exponential elimination from a single compartment is

$$\frac{d\,(mC)}{dt} = If_w - k\,(mC) \tag{5.5}$$

or,

time rate of change of mass of element in organ = (rate of uptake from ingestion) − (rate of elimination)

Figure 5.1 illustrates a single compartment model. Integrating (5.5) gives:

$$mC = \frac{If_w}{k}\,(1 - e^{-kt}) \tag{5.6}$$

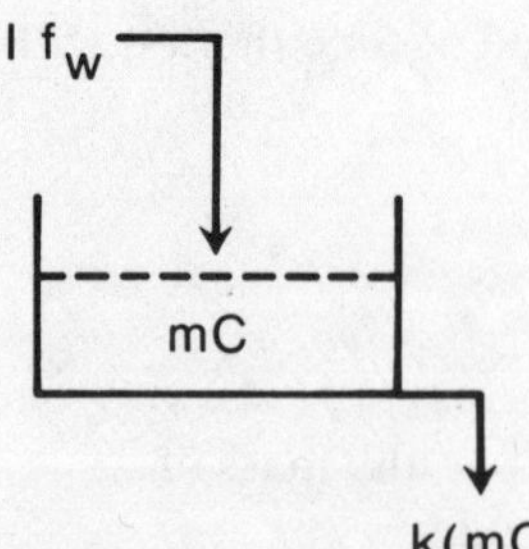

Figure 5.1. Single compartment model schematic.

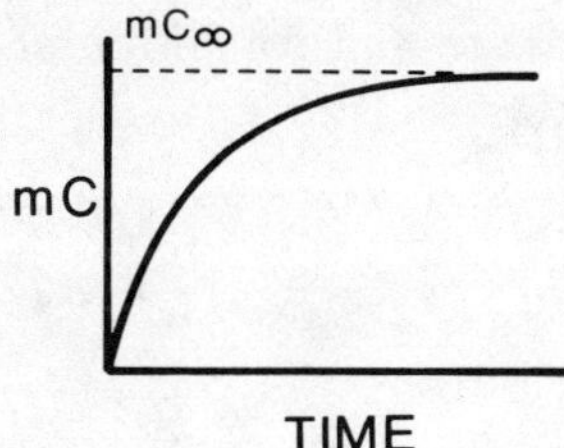

Figure 5.2. Change in body burden with time for continuous exposure at a constant concentration.

where t is time of exposure. Substituting the definition of k into (5.6) gives:

$$mC = \frac{If_w T_b}{0.693}(1 - e^{-0.693\, t/T_b}) \tag{5.7}$$

Furthermore, if $t/T_b >> 1$, then equilibrium between uptake and elimination exists,

$$\frac{d(mC)}{dt} = 0$$

and

$$mC_\infty = \frac{If_w T_b}{0.693} \tag{5.8}$$

Where C_∞ is the equilibrium mass ratio.

Figure 5.2 is a plot of (5.7). For inhalation instead of ingestion replace f_w by f_a in (5.7) and (5.8). For insoluble material in the lung T_b = 120 days (except for plutonium for which T_b = 1 year and thorium for which T_b = 4 years) (1); for radioactive material replace T_b with T_e.

Example of Continuous Intake of a Constant Concentration

Assume an individual is ingesting water that contains 10 μg/liter of lead and that the following values are applicable, assuming bone as the critical organ (1,2):

$$\begin{aligned} \text{mass of total body} &= 7 \times 10^4\text{g} \\ \text{mass of bone} &= 7 \times 10^3\text{g} \\ \text{biological half-life } T_b &= 3.65 \times 10^3 \text{ days (bone)} \\ f_w &= 0.02 \\ f_a &= 0.08 \end{aligned}$$

(Note that values of f_w and f_a may vary with dosage and for different compounds of the same element).

For ingestion

$$mC_\infty = \frac{If_wT_b}{0.693}$$

water intake = 2.2 liter/day

$$I = 10\ \mu\text{g/liter} \times 2.2\ \text{liter/day} = 22\ \mu\text{g/day}$$

Therefore

$$mC_\infty = \frac{(22\ \mu\text{g/day})\ (0.02)\ (3.65 \times 10^3\ \text{days})}{0.693}$$

$$mC_\infty = 2.32 \times 10^3\ \mu\text{g} = 2.32\ \text{mg from water}$$

If, in addition, the individual is inhaling air with a lead concentration of 3 μg/m^3 the organ (bone) burden from inhalation will be

$$mC_\infty = \frac{If_aT_b}{0.693}$$

air inhaled = 20 m^3/day

$$I = 3\ \mu\text{g/m}^3 \times 20\ \text{m}^3\text{/day} = 60\ \mu\text{g/day}$$

and,

$$mC_\infty = \frac{(60\ \mu\text{g/day})\ (0.08)\ (3.65 \times 10^3\text{days})}{0.693}$$

$$mC_\infty = 25.3 \times 10^3\ \mu\text{g} = 25.3\ \text{mg from air}$$

$$\begin{aligned} mC_\infty &= \text{total bone burden at equilibrium} \\ &= mC_\infty\ (\text{air}) + mC_\infty\ (\text{water}) = 25.3 + 2.32 = 27.6\ \text{mg lead} \end{aligned}$$

This value represents about 90% of the whole-body burden.

Single Intake

The single intake model can be described by

$$mC_0 = A_0f_w\ \text{(for ingestion) or}\ A_0f_a\ \text{(for inhalation)} \tag{5.9}$$

or,

initial mass of element in organ	=	(amount ingested or inhaled) (fraction of the amount ingested or inhaled deposited in the critical organ)

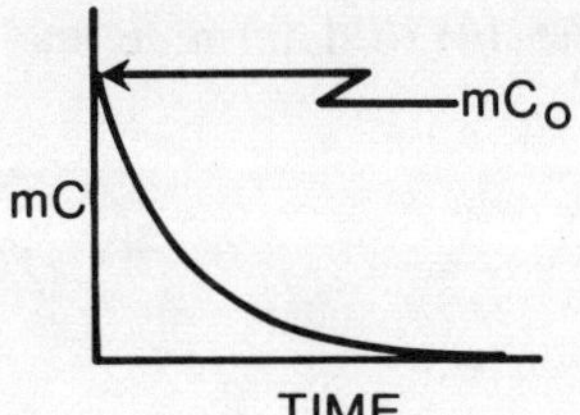

Figure 5.3. Exponential elimination for a single intake body burden model.

where

C_0 = concentration of element initially in organ ($t = 0$)
A_0 = mass of the single intake ingested or inhaled

For single compartment exponential elimination the mass of element in the organ will decrease exponentially. This relationship is shown in Figure 5.3 and can be expressed as

$$mC = mC_0 e^{-kt} \tag{5.10}$$

where

t = time after exposure

Examples of Single Intakes

Ingestion

Assume that an individual ingests 100 μg of lead (e.g., by drinking from a lead-glazed cup). The amount deposited in the bone would be

$$mC_0 = A_0 f_w = 100\ \mu\text{g}\ (0.02) = 2\ \mu\text{g of lead}$$

Inhalation

Assume an individual inhales air containing 100 μg/m³ of lead for 1 hr at a breathing rate of 10 m³ for 8 hr. Then

$$A_0 = 100\ \mu\text{g/m}^3 \times \frac{10\ \text{m}^0}{8\ \text{hr}} \times 1\ \text{hr} = 125\ \mu\text{g}$$

and

$$mC_0 = (125)\ (0.08) = 10\ \mu\text{g of lead}$$

These values of mC_0 can then be substituted in (5.10) to determine lead retention at any time after exposure.

MULTICOMPARTMENTAL MODELS

The body burden models discussed previously serve as a starting point to understanding the kinetics involved in the intake, uptake, and elimination of environmental pollutants. These are very simplified and, as such, generally serve as imprecise predictors of body burdens in specific individuals. The estimates are useful when evaluating potential impact on large numbers of individuals at risk to environmental stressors.

Both (5.6) and (5.10) assume a single compartment and exponential elimination. Multicompartmental models provide a better fit to actual animal and human data. For example, a three-compartment model (blood, soft tissue, and bone) has been developed for lead metabolism in normal adults (6,7). A two-compartment model describing uptake and excretion kinetics has been proposed for humans exposed to atmospheric lead (8). Animal studies have provided data on the excretion of lead based upon an exponential model with four compartments (blood and internal organs representing rapid exchange; skin and muscles; the exchangeable part of lead in bones; and the very slowly exchanged part of lead in bone) (4).

The retention of lead, as well as many other bone-seeking elements, may be more satisfactorily treated as a power function rather than as an exponential (4)

$$R_t = At^{-n} \tag{5.11}$$

where,

R_t = retention of lead at time t as a function of dose
A = retention at $t = 1$
n = coefficient of rate of loss from the body

Although some of these multicompartmental models may prove to be useful, there is great difficulty at the present time in obtaining suitable data for their validation. For example, the relationships between lead in blood, urine, and critical organs (e.g., bone marrow, which is useful to characterize chronic exposure) are not well defined because of the passive nature of bone lead compared to the active (readily exchanged) lead in tissue. Samples of cortical bone would be preferable for estimating total whole-body burden. Since such specimens are not readily available, other samples (blood, urine, hair, teeth) must be used. However, none of these are as valid indicators of whole-body burden resulting from long-time exposure as cortical bone (9).

Consequently, multicompartmental models are useful in analyzing the specifics of pollutant uptake and elimination. However, the data necessary to use them for environmental evaluations are presently not available for most pollutants.

REFERENCES

1. International Commission on Radiation Protection. *Report of Committee II on Permissible Dose for Internal Radiation*. ICRP Publication No. 2, Pergamon Press, New York, 1960.
2. International Commission on Radiation Protection. *Report of the Task Group on Reference Man*. ICRP Publication No. 23, Pergamon Press, New York, 1975.
3. Task Group on Lung Dynamics. Deposition and retention models for internal dosimetry of the human respiratory tract. *Health Phys.* **12**:173–208, 1966.
4. Task Group on Metal Accumulation. Accumulation of toxic metals with special reference to their absorption, excretion, and biological half-time. *Environ. Physiol. Biochem.* **3**:65–107, 1973.
5. International Committee on Radiation Protection. *The Assessment of Internal Contamination Resulting from Recurrent or Prolonged Uptakes*. ICRP Publication No. 10A, Pergamon Press, New York, 1971.
6. Rabinowitz, M. B., Wetherill, G. W., and Kopple, J. D. Kinetic analysis of lead metabolism in healthy humans. *J. Clin. Invest.* **58**:260–270, 1976.
7. Rabinowitz, M. B., Wetherill, G. W., and Kopple, J. D. Magnitude of lead intake from respiration by normal man. *J. Clin. Invest.* **58**:238–248, 1977.
8. Knelson, J. H., Johnson, R. J., Coulston, F., Goldberg, L., and Griffin, T. Kinetics of respiratory lead uptake in humans. *Proceedings of the International Symposium on Environmental Health Aspects of Lead.* Commission of the European Communities—U.S. Environmental Protection Agency, Amsterdam, 1972.
9. Environmental Health Resource Center. *Environmental Lead: Health Effects and Recommended Standards*. Illinois Institute for Environmental Quality Document No. EHRC-1, November 1972, pp. 1–22 (distributed as PB220-224 by the National Technical Information Service).

[illegible]

[illegible]

[illegible]

[illegible]

6

PHYSIOLOGICAL CHANGES

William H. Hallenbeck, William H. Kojola, and Sally J. Jansen

Until recently an environmental pollutant was not considered a threat to human health unless its concentration was high enough to produce an observable disease syndrome, that is, a clinical effect. Recent evidence has shown that relatively small physiological changes are often produced by low concentrations of environmental pollutants. Physiological changes that do not produce an observable disease syndrome are referred to as subclinical effects. These effects range from subtle changes in blood chemistry or lung function, which may be reversible, to small changes in the nervous tissue, which may be irreversible and permanent. An important characteristic of a subclinical effect is that it is usually below human perception and can only be detected by biochemical or physiological tests. However, such effects do represent interruption of normal physiological processes.

Subclinical effects raise at least two important health questions. Even though a healthy person does not perceive a pollutant-induced subclinical effect, is there a cumulative effect from chronic low-level exposure that may result in a clinical effect? Little is known about this question and much research is needed. Second, are there hypersusceptible human population groups for whom a small physiological change may trigger a clinical reaction? There is evidence that clearly indicates that certain groups react adversely to concentrations of pollutants that do not perceptibly affect healthy persons. Individuals with pulmonary disease and those with cardiovascular dysfunction are at high risk to ambient levels of environmental pollutants.

Many variables enter into the process of planning new energy producing and using facilities. The health implications of the facility for hypersusceptible population groups deserve special consideration. In addition, as research provides more information, it may become important to consider the effect of long-term exposure to pollutant concentrations that produce subclinical effects in healthy persons.

Carbon monoxide, ozone, and lead are three pollutants that produce subclinical effects. The following discussion of these pollutants illustrates the nature of the low-level physiological changes that they produce in healthy and hypersusceptible groups.

PHYSIOLOGICAL CHANGES DUE TO CARBON MONOXIDE

Exposure to carbon monoxide (CO) in the environment or workplace results in physiological changes that reduce the oxygen-carrying capacity of the blood. Depending on the ambient concentration of CO, the length of exposure, and individual susceptibility, these physiological changes may result in either subclinical or clinical health effects.

Carbon monoxide diffuses rapidly across the alveolar membranes in the lung and binds reversibly with hemoglobin (Hb) in the red blood cells to form carboxyhemoglobin (COHb). The affinity of Hb for CO is 200–250 times that for oxygen (O_2) (1). In addition to COHb formation, exposure to CO causes O_2 to bond more tightly with the remaining Hb. The increased tightness of the oxyhemoglobin (HBO_2) bond means that tissue oxygen must fall to lower than normal levels before HbO_2 gives up its O_2 (2).

A theoretical equation (the CFK equation) has been developed that relates exposure to CO to percent COHb saturation (3). Data obtained from human exposure studies strongly support this model (4,5). Figure 6.1 is based on solutions of the CFK equation.

The presence of CO in the human body originates from endogenous and exogenous sources. Normal breakdown of Hb produces a low concentration of endogenous CO which results in a COHb saturation of 0.3–0.7%.

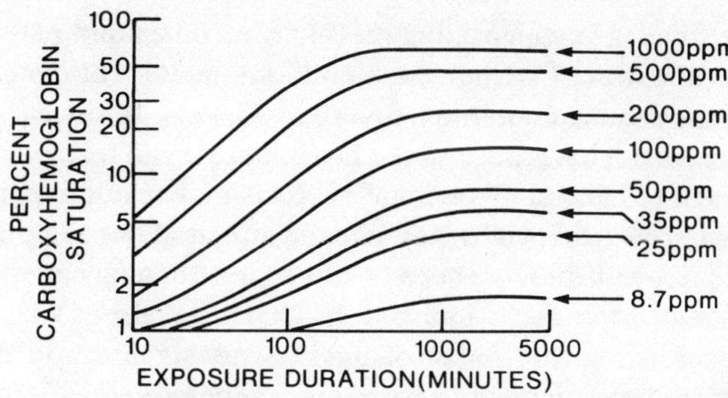

Figure 6.1. Carboxyhemoglobin levels for man as a function of exposure duration and CO concentration as determined by solving the CFK equation [from (3,5)]. Values of all parameters other than CO were nominal and held constant: P_B = barometric pressure = 750 mm Hg; $\bar{P}_{C_{O_2}}$ = average partial pressure of oxygen in lung capillaries = 100 mm Hg; $\dot{V}_A$ = alveolar ventilation rate = 6000 ml/min; M = ratio of the affinity of blood for CO to that for O_2 = 218; V_b = blood volume = 5500 ml; $D_{L_{CO}}$ = diffusivity of the lung for CO = 30 ml/min-mm Hg; $\{COHb\}_0$ = blood CO at the beginning of the exposure level = 0.8%; and $\dot{V}_{CO}$ = rate of endogenous CO production = 0.007 ml/min.

Disease states may contribute to endogenous CO production. For example, patients with hemolytic anemia may have a COHb saturation of 4–6% (1).

Exogenous sources of CO are usually associated with the incomplete combustion of carbonaceous material. Tobacco smokers are the most heavily exposed nonindustrial group and may have a COHb saturation of 6–9% (1). The increased COHb levels caused by smoking cigarettes have been shown to decrease the rate of oxygen delivery to heart tissue with subsequent reduction in the ability to exercise before onset of anginal pain (6). Motor vehicle exhaust accounts for about 80% of environmental CO emissions. Peak-hour traffic can generate levels of 25 ppm of CO which, during inversions, may rise to 100 ppm. Fuel combustion at stationary sources, industrial process discharges, and solid waste disposal account for another 20% of the total emissions of CO (1).

Myocardial (heart muscle) tissue has a high demand for O_2. At rest 75% of the O_2 is extracted from the coronary circulation as compared to 25% in peripheral tissue. Normally, increased myocardial demand for O_2 is met by increasing the flow rate of coronary circulation. Consequently a healthy person is able to adapt to a modest increase in COHb. However, coronary vascular disease may prevent an increase in blood flow to compensate for stresses such as COHb, a tightened HbO_2 bond, and exercise (2,7). In this event an alternative compensating mechanism comes into play. Myocardial tissue will extract O_2 from the blood at a greater rate; increased O_2 extraction may reduce O_2 in the blood to low levels. If low enough blood levels are reached, some areas of the heart muscle will be oxygen starved and subclinical to clinical myocardial necrosis may result in persons with heart disease. The effects of a 90-min exposure at about 53 ppm of CO in Los Angeles freeway air have been observed in 10 angina patients (7). The subjects developed a mean increase in COHb levels of 4%, and their ability to exercise before onset of angina was significantly decreased. Average COHb levels increased from 1 to 5% before and after exposure. It has also been demonstrated that a mean increase in COHb of only 1.6% can cause significantly decreased exercise tolerance in persons with stable angina pectoris; 10 patients were exposed to 50 ppm of CO under laboratory conditions for 4 hr (8). Average COHb levels increased from 1.3 to 2.9% before and after exposure to CO. In another study 10 patients with exertional angina pectoris were exposed to 50 ppm CO for 2 hr under laboratory conditions (9). A mean increase in COHb of 1.7% caused significantly decreased exercise tolerance. Average COHb levels increased from 1.0 to 2.7% before and after exposure.

Table 6.1 lists some of the known subclinical and clinical physiological responses to CO exposure. Whether clinical or subclinical health effects follow exposure to ambient CO depends largely on individual susceptibility. The following groups are hypersusceptible to the toxic effects of CO: heavy smokers, infants, and persons with cardiovascular disease, anemia, lung disease, and increased metabolic rate (1). Individuals with hemolytic anemia or who are heavy smokers will have elevated COHb levels before exposure to ambient CO. Persons with severe heart disease may not possess sufficient cardiac reserve to compensate for CO exposures to which healthy members of the population can adapt.

PHYSIOLOGICAL CHANGES DUE TO OZONE

Ozone is one of the major environmental air pollutants present in the ambient atmosphere, with concentrations ranging from less than 0.02 ppm to greater than 0.60 ppm in the urban environment (10). It is recognized as a bronchopulmonary irritant that adversely affects lung tissue and parameters of lung function (11). When inhaled it initiates biochemical changes in the blood (12). While ambient levels of ozone have not, as yet, been

Table 6.1 Human Response to Various Carboxyhemoglobin Levels (1)

CO (ppm)	Time of exposure (hours)	COHB Saturation (%)	Response of Healthy Adult	Response of Patient with Severe Heart Disease (Hypersusceptible)
		0.3–0.7	Endogenous CO production. No known detrimental effect.	
		1.5	Increase in blood flow to certain vital organs such as the heart.	May lack sufficient cardiac reserve to compensate.
50	1.5–4	2.7–5.1	Visual light threshold increased.	Less exertion required to induce pain in patients with angina pectoris (7–9).
		16–20	Headache; visual evoked response abnormal.	May be lethal.
		20–30	Throbbing headache; nausea; fine manual dexterity abnormal.	
		30–40	Severe headache; nausea and vomiting; syncope.	
		50	Coma; convulsions.	
		67–70	Lethal if not treated.	

linked with increases in mortality or production of disease states in humans (11), there is evidence that these levels may result in physiological and biochemical changes that constitute subclinical effects.

Perturbations in several parameters of human lung function are the predominant known subclinical effects resulting from ozone inhalation. Table 6.2 summarizes subclinical changes in lung function following ozone exposure and indicates the level of exposure, the type of subject exposed (normal or hypersusceptible), whether exercise was performed, and the number of parameters showing statistically significant change in pulmonary function. Significant changes in lung function generally begin to appear at 0.25 ppm after 2 to 4-hr exposures (13,14). Significant subclinical lung function changes also occur as ozone concentrations increase from 0.37 to 0.90 ppm (13–19). The health significance of such changes in lung function is presently not well understood.

Subclinical biochemical changes in blood also occur in humans following ozone inhalation. Exposure to 0.25 ppm produced few or no important biochemical changes (14). However, upon exposure to 0.37–0.40 ppm, biochemical analysis revealed statistically significant decreases in red blood cell acetylcholinesterase activity and reduced glutathione levels, along with increases in red cell glucose-6-phosphate dehydrogenase and lactate dehydrogenase activities (14,20).

Exposure to 0.50 ppm not only demonstrated biochemical changes identical and generally more severe than those found at 0.37–0.40 ppm but, in addition, showed statistically significant increases in red cell membrane fragility, serum vitamin E levels, and lipid peroxidation, as well as decreases in hemoglobin and hematocrit values (12,20–22). Such alterations disappear gradually, and some are still detectable two weeks after inhalation. The health significance of these subclinical alterations in blood biochemistry is currently unknown.

PHYSIOLOGICAL CHANGES DUE TO LEAD

Although cases of clinical lead poisoning in children and workers remain a problem today, the question of subclinical physiological effects at low levels of exposure is of increasing concern. Lead can interfere with the biosynthesis of heme. (Heme is the precursor of hemoglobin, which is the O_2-carrying substance in the blood.) The points at which inhibition occurs in this pathway are indicated in Figure 6.2 (23). Because of the inhibition

Table 6.2 Subclinical Changes in Pulmonary Function of Humans Exposed to Ozone in Environmental Chambers

Ozone Concentration (ppm)	Duration of Exposure	Number and Type of Subjects[a]	Exercise[b]	Number of Parameters of Pulmonary Function Tested[c]	Number of Parameters Showing Significant Change in Pulmonary Function[d]	Reference
0.25	2 hr	7 N and H	yes	12	3	14
0.25	4 hr	4 H	no	14	1	13
0.37	2 hr	5 N and H	yes	13	1	14
0.37	2 hr	12 N	yes	4	4	15
0.37	4 hr	4 H	no	14	4	13
0.50	2 hr	7 N and H	yes	13	10	14
0.50	4 hr	4 N	no	14	5	13
0.50	4 hr	4 H	no	14	7	13
0.60	2 hr	24 N	yes	3	3	16
0.60–0.80	2 hr	11 N	no	6	3	17
0.75	2 hr	12 N	yes	4	4	15
0.75	2 hr	10 N	no	9	3	18
0.90	5 min	4 N	yes	1	1	19

[a] N = Normal subjects, e.g., subjects with no history of cough, chest discomfort, wheezing, allergy, or respiratory disease; H = hypersusceptible subjects, e.g., subjects with a history of cough, chest discomfort, wheezing, or allergy.

[b] Brisk walking or riding bicycle ergometer.

[c] Includes forced vital capacity, forced expiratory volume, total respiratory resistance, closing volume, airway resistance, lung compliance, diffusing capacity, vital capacity, maximal midexpiratory flow rate, maximum static elastic recoil pressure, specific airway conductance.

[d] $P \leqslant .05$. P = probability of control-exposure difference being due to chance.

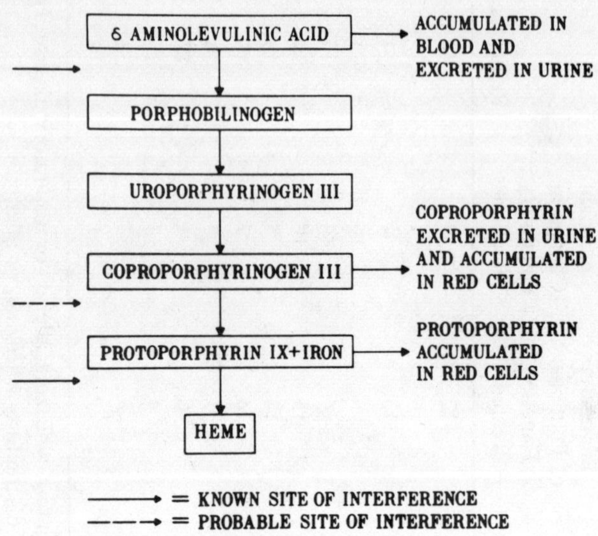

Figure 6.2. Biosynthesis of heme. From "Lead Poisoning," J. J. Chisolm, Jr.

of enzymes involved in the biosynthesis of heme, metabolites accumulate in the blood and urine, for example, free erythrocyte protoporphyrin (FEP), erythrocyte zinc protoporphyrin (ZPP), free erythrocyte coproporphyrin, urinary coproporphyrin, and δ-aminolevulinic acid (ALA). Changes in the levels of several physiological indicators have been used to estimate increased human exposure to lead: increases in FEP, ZPP, free erythrocyte coproporphyrin, urinary coproporphyrin, ALA, and lead in whole blood (PbB); decreases in δ-aminolevulinic acid dehydratase (ALAD) activity, and peripheral nerve conduction velocity. Four of these indices (PbB, ALAD, FEP, and nerve conduction velocity) are discussed below.

Until recently blood lead was the most widely used biological indicator of lead exposure. Four ranges of PbB concentrations are usually considered to indicate the following conditions (24):

1. "Normal": mean $\simeq$ 20 μg/100 ml; range 5–40 μg/100 ml.
2. Undue absorption: $>$ 40 μg/100 ml.
3. Increased lead absorption: 50–80 μg/100 ml.
4. Clearly evident clinical lead poisoning: usually associated with concentrations $>$ 80 μg/100 ml.

The inhibition of ALAD activity in red blood cells is the most sensitive biological manifestation of exposure to lead. There is a negative relationship (Figure 6.3) between PbB and ALAD (25–27). Some studies suggest that there is a no-effect level at 10–15 μg (PbB)/100 ml (28,29), while others indicate the ALAD is inhibited at any level of PbB (25,30,31). The biological significance of ALAD inhibition is uncertain. However, since ALAD is required for hemoglobin synthesis, for the formation of a number of heme-containing respiratory enzymes, and is also present in a large number of tissues (31), it is likely that ALAD inhibition has health significance.

Increased lead burden interferes with iron utilization and results in the accumulation of protoporphyrin in erythrocytes, excess iron in the blood, and ultimately anemia. The elevation may persist for months, even after blood lead has decreased considerably (28). Protoporphyrins are measured as FEP or ZPP. There is a positive correlation between log FEP and PbB (Figure 6.3). Threshold values for the FEP response have been observed at 20 μg (PbB)/100 ml for children (25). Other studies have found thresholds of response to be 20–25 μg (PbB)/100 ml for adult females and children, and 25–30 μg (PbB)/100 ml for adult males (28).

A further illustration of subclinical effects is provided by evidence of peripheral nerve damage in workers and children. The effect of lead exposure on the peripheral nervous system was investigated in workers with no clinical symptoms and whose blood leads never exceeded 70 μg/100 ml (32). The main findings were the statistically significant slowing of motor nerve conduction velocities in the forearm (median and ulnar nerves). Electromyographical abnormalities were also observed. The well-being of these workers did not seem to be influenced by the neuropathy; however, the investigators regarded subclinical neuropathy as a more serious effect than the reversible alterations in heme synthesis because the nervous system has a poor regenerative capacity. Similar findings have been noted in children. A study of children, all apparently healthy, living near a primary lead smelter in Idaho revealed a statistically significant inverse relationship between PbB and motor nerve conduction velocity in 5–9 year-olds. None of the children had clinical neurologic disease or clearly pathologic conduction velocities (33).

Several population subgroups may be hypersusceptible to the effects of lead exposure. Young children are more susceptible than adults because of their immature physiological development, especially of the central nervous system (34). The tendency to place nonfood substances in their

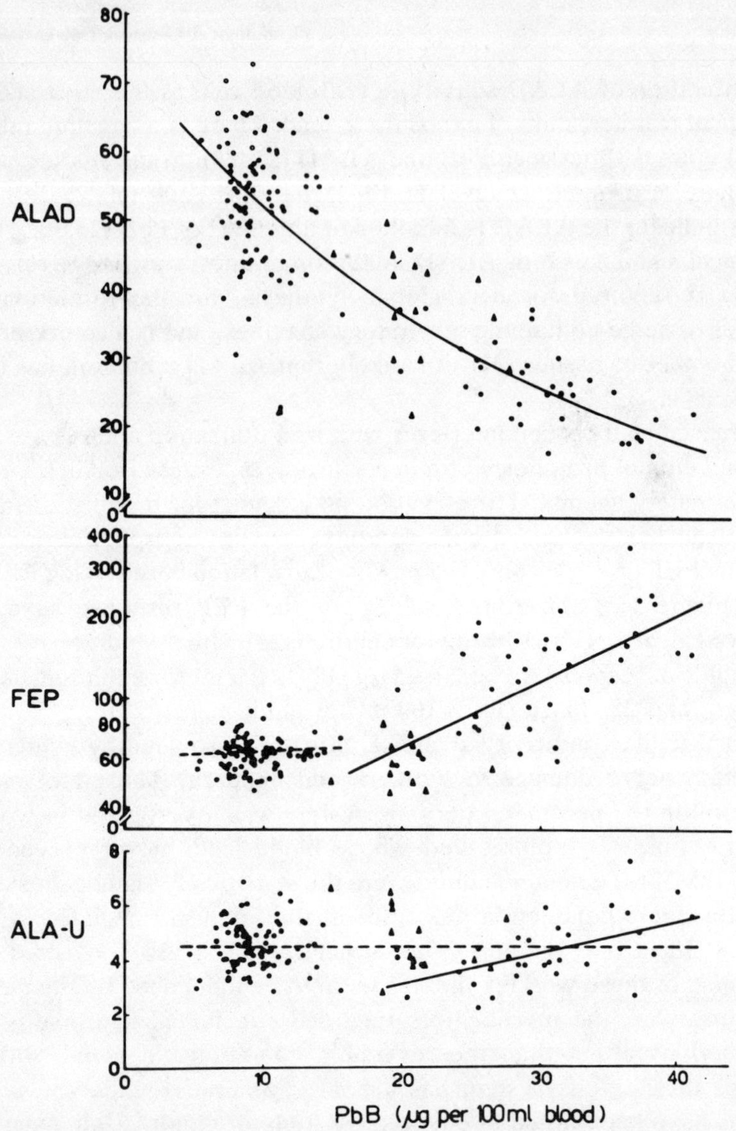

Figure 6.3. Relationships between lead concentration in blood (PbB) and three biological measurements in children: ALAD (δ-aminolevulinic acid dehydratase activity expressed in nmol δ-aminolevulinic acid transformed/min/ml erythrocytes); FEP (free erythrocyte prophyrin expressed in μg/100 ml erythrocytes), and ALAU (δ-aminolevulinic acid in urine expressed in mg/g creatinine). *Open circles,* rural children; *solid circles,* children living less than 1 km from lead smelter; *triangles,* children living 2.5 km from lead smelter. *Dotted line:* FEP, regression line for rural children ($N = 92$); ALAU, regression line for total child population ($N = 143$). *Solid line:* ALAD, regression line for total child population ($N = 143$); FEP, regression line for children living in lead smelter area ($N = 51$); ALAU, regression line for children living less than 1 km from lead smelter ($N = 37$) [from (25)].

mouths makes children more likely to be exposed to lead in paint, soil, and dust. Furthermore, one study suggests that the rate of intestinal absorption and retention of lead is greater in children than in adults (35). As increasing numbers of women enter the workplace attention is being focused on the abortifacient effects of lead (36). In addition the level of FEP in women and children appears to increase at a greater rate (as a function of PbB) than in males (25). Certain medical conditions may increase susceptibility to the effects of lead. These include iron deficiency states or disorders characterized by impairment of iron utilization (such as copper deficiency, vitamin B_6 deficiency, and thalassemia) (37).

REFERENCES

1. Stewart, R. D. The effect of carbon monoxide on humans. *J. Occup. Med.* **18**:304–309, 1976.
2. Ayres, S. M., Mueller, H. S., Gregory, J. J., Giannelli, S., and Penny, J. L. Systemic and myocardial hemodynamic responses to relatively small concentrations of carboxyhemoglobin (COHb). *Arch. Environ. Health.* **18**:699–709, 1969.
3. Coburn, R. F., Forster, R. E., and Kane, P. B. Considerations of the physiological variables that determine the blood carboxyhemoglobin concentration in man. *J. Clin. Invest.* **44**:1899–1910, 1965.
4. Peterson, J. E. and Stewart, R. D. Absorption and Elimination of carbon monoxide by inactive young men. *Arch. Environ. Health.* **21**:165–171, 1970.
5. Peterson, J. E. and Stewart, R. D. Predicting the carboxyhemoglobin levels resulting from carbon monoxide exposures. *J. Appl. Physiol.* **39**:622–638, 1975.
6. Aronow, W. S. and Rokay S. N. Carboxyhemoglobin caused by smoking nonnicotine cigarettes. Effects in angina pectoris. *Circulation.* **44**:782–788, 1971.
7. Aronow, W. S., Harris, C. N., Isbell, M. W., Rokay, S. N., and Imparato, B. Effect of freeway travel on angina pectoris. *Ann. Intern. Med.* **77**:669–676, 1972.
8. Anderson, E. W., Andelman, R. J., Strauch, J. M., Fortuin, N. J., and Knelson, J. H. Effect of low-level carbon monoxide exposure on onset and duration of angina pectoris. *Ann. Intern. Med.* **9**:46–50, 1973.
9. Aronow, W. S. and Isbell, M. W. Carbon monoxide effect on exercise-induced angina pectoris. *Ann. Intern. Med.* **79**:392–395, 1973.
10. U.S. Department of Health, Education, and Welfare. Public Health Service. National Air Pollution Control Administration. *Air Quality Criteria for Photochemical Oxidants.* NAPCA Publ. No. AP-63. Washington, DC, 1970.

11. National Academy of Sciences. National Research Council. Committee on Medical and Biologic Effects of Environmental Pollutants, *Ozone and Other Photochemical Oxidants*. Washington, DC, 1977.
12. Buckley, R. D., Hackney, J. D., Clark, K., and Posin, C. Ozone and human blood. *Arch. Environ. Health.* **30**:40–43, 1975.
13. Hackney, J. D., Linn, W. S., Mohler, J. G., Pederson, E. E., Breisacher, P., and Russo, A. Experimental studies on human health effects of air pollutants. II. Four-hour exposure to ozone alone and in combination with other pollutant gases. *Arch. Environ. Health.* **30**:379–384, 1975.
14. Hackney, J. D., Linn, W. S., Law, D. C., Karuza, S. K., Greenberg, H., Buckley, R. D., and Pederson, E. E. Experimental studies on human health effects of air pollutants. III. Two-hour exposure to ozone alone and in combination with other pollutant gases. *Arch. Environ. Health.* **30**:385–390, 1975.
15. Hazucha, M., Silverman, F., Parent, C., Field, S., and Bates, D. V. Pulmonary function in man after short-term exposure to ozone. *Arch. Environ. Health.* **27**:183–188, 1973.
16. Ketcham, B. T., Lassiter, S., Haak, E. D., and Knelson, J. H. Ozone exposure impairs pulmonary function in healthy young men. *Clin. Res.* **25**:37A, 1977.
17. Young, W. A., Shaw, D. B., and Bates, D. V. Effect of low concentrations of ozone on pulmonary function in man. *J. Appl. Physiol.* **19**:765–768, 1964.
18. Bates, D. V., Bell, G. M., Burnham, C. D., Hazucha, M., Mantha, J., Pengelly, L. D., and Silverman, F. Short-term effects of ozone on the lung. *J. Appl. Physiol.* **32**:176–181, 1972.
19. Kagawa, J. and Toyama, T. Effects of ozone and brief exercise on specific airway conductance in man. *Arch. Environ. Health.* **30**:36–39, 1975.
20. Buckley, R. D., Hackney, J. D., Clark, K., and Posin, C. Biochemical changes in human blood following ozone inhalation. *Environ. Health Perspect.* **16**:185, 1976.
21. Buckley, R. D., Hackney, J. D., Clark, K., and Posin, C. Some effects of ozone inhalation on human erythrocyte metabolism. *Fed. Proc.* **33**:335, 1974.
22. Buckley, R., Hackney, J., Clark, K., and Posin, C. Erythrocyte biochemistry in humans exposed to ozone. *Fed. Proc.* **36**:630, 1977.
23. Chisolm, J. J. Lead poisoning. *Sci. Am.* **224**:15–23, 1971.
24. Chisolm, J. J. Screening techniques for undue lead exposure in children: biological and practical considerations. *J. Pediatr.* **79**:719–725, 1971.
25. Roels, H., Buchet, J., Lauwerys, R., Hubermont, G., Bruaux, P., Claeys-Thoreau, F., LaFontaine, A., and Van Overschelde, J. Impact of air pollution by lead on the heme biosynthetic pathway in school-age children. *Arch. Environ. Health.* **31**:310–317, 1976.
26. Wada, O., Takeo, K., Yano, Y., Ono, T., Nagahashi, M., and Seki, H. δ-Aminolevulinic acid dehydratase in low level exposure. *Arch. Environ. Health.* **31**:211–214, 1976.

27. Weissberg, J., Lipschutz, F., and Oski, F. δ-Aminolevulinic acid dehydratase activity in circulating blood cells. *N. Engl. J. Med.* **284**:565–569, 1971.

28. Zielhuis, R. L. Dose-response relationships for inorganic lead. *Int. Arch. Occup. Health.* **35**:1–18, 1975.

29. Granick, J. L., Sassa, S., Granick, S., Levere, R. D., and Kappas, A. Studies in lead poisoning. II. Correlation between the ratio of activated to inactivated δ-aminolevulinic acid dehydratase of whole blood and blood lead level. *Biochem. Med.* **8**:149–159, 1973.

30. Hernberg, S. and Nikkanen, J. Enzyme inhibition by lead under normal urban conditions. *Lancet.* **1**:63–64, 1970.

31. Hernberg, S. Biological effects of low lead doses. In *Proceedings International Symposium Environmental Health Aspects of Lead.* Commission of European Communities and U.S. Environmental Protection Agency, 1973, pp. 617–629.

32. Seppalainen, A., Sakari, T., Hernberg, S., and Kock, B. Subclinical neuropathy at "safe" levels of lead exposure. *Arch. Environ. Health.* **30**:180–183, 1975.

33. Landrigan, P. J., Baker, E. L., Feldman, R. G., Cox, D. H., Eden, K. V., Orenstein, W. A., Mather, J. A., Yankel, A. J., and Von Lindern, I. H. Increased lead absorption with anemia and slowed nerve conduction in children near a lead smelter. *J. Pediatr.* **89**:904–910, 1976.

34. Waldron, H. A. and Stofen, D. *Subclinical Lead Poisoning.* Academic Press, Inc. New York, 1974.

35. Alexander, F. W., Delves, H. T., and Clayton, B. E. The uptake and excretion by children of lead and other contaminants. In *Proceedings International Symposium Environmental Health Aspects of Lead.* Commission of European Communities and U.S. Environmental Protection Agency, 1973, pp. 319–332.

36. Rom, W. N. Effects of lead on the female and reproduction: A Review. *Mt. Sinai J. Med.* **43**:542–552, 1976.

37. National Academy of Science. *Airborne Lead in Perspective.* Committee on Biological Effects of Atmospheric Pollutants. Division of Medical Sciences, National Research Council, Washington, DC, 1972.

CHARACTERIZATION OF ENVIRONMENTAL HAZARDS

7

IDENTIFICATION AND QUANTITATION OF STRESSORS

Richard A. Wadden

Incorporation of health considerations into project planning begins with identification of the potential health hazards that may be discharged. Evaluation can be roughly divided into three major areas: what goes into the process, what the process is supposed to do, and how the process is operated. As an example, the basic physical-chemical structure of the coal fed to fossil-fueled power plants results in greater amounts of carcinogenic polycyclic hydrocarbons in the stack gas than the amounts that result from burning an equivalent quantity of natural gas (1) (Figure 7.1).

What the process is supposed to do and how it is operated may be two quite different considerations. When operating continuously under steady conditions the carbon monoxide emissions from an auto exhaust pipe are typically only 10–20% of the emissions from the same engine initially starting up (2). The same is true of many chemical and energy processes where start-up emissions, due to nonsteady-state operating conditions of temperature, pressure, and flow, are much in excess of those during design operation. Sulfuric acid plants require certain process components

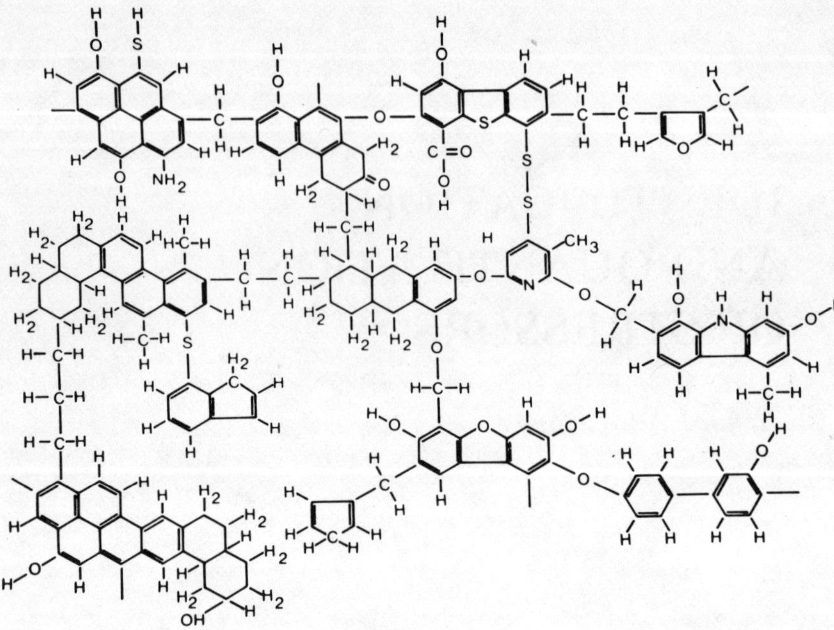

Figure 7.1. A representative bituminous coal structure (3).

to operate at temperatures up to 1150°F. When starting up such plants, 6–24 hr may be required to heat all the equipment to design temperatures. Unless proper control measures are instituted the discharge of sulfuric acid mist and sulphur dioxide (SO_2) will be much greater than under steady-state conditions. Finally, the most sophisticated control device in existence still depends on a man to turn it on (or off) and maintain it.

After identification of hazardous materials, the amounts and potential environmental release rates must be quantitated. Information is available for pollutants like particulates and nitrogen oxides for such things as new automobiles and oil-fired power plants (2). Table 7.1 gives a set of emission factors that can be used to estimate emissions from such power plants based on the amount of fuel burned. The data is harder to come by for: (1) less commonly considered pollutants, such as benzo(a)pyrene from coal combustion; (2) new, untested technologies, such as coal gasification; and (3) older, existing pollution sources, such as diesel buses and trucks that have been poorly maintained. Amounts of a particular pollutant discharged to air, water, and soil must be measured or estimated.

Table 7.1 Emission Factors for Fuel Oil Combustion (2)

	Unit: Industrial and Commercial							
	Power Plant		Residual		Distillate		Domestic	
Pollutant	lb/10^3 gal	kg/10^3 liters	lb/10^3 gal	kg/10^3 liters	lb/10^3 gal	kg/10^3 liters	lb/10^3 gal	kg/10^3 liters
Particulate	8	1	23	2.75	15	1.8	10	1.2
Sulfur dioxide[a]	157S	19S	157S	19S	142S	17S	142S	17S
Sulfur trioxide[a]	2S	0.25S	2S	0.25S	2S	0.25S	2S	0.25S
Carbon monoxide	3	0.4	4	0.5	4	0.5	5	0.6
Hydrocarbons	2	0.25	3	0.35	3	0.35	3	0.35
Nitrogen oxides (NO_2)	105	12.6	(40–80)	(4.8–9.6)	(40–80)	(4.8–9.6)	12	1.5
Aldehydes (HCHO)	1	0.12	1	0.12	2	0.25	2	0.25

[a] S = percent by weight of sulfur in the oil.

Table 7.2 Some Trace Elements in Coal and Coal Gasifier Gas (3)

	Concentration (lb of trace element/ 1000 tons of coal)	
Element	Coal	Coal Gasifier Gas
As	28.0	27.7
B	204	97.3
Be	3.2	0.1
Cd	5.0	
Co	19.1	
Cr	27.5	
Cu	30.3	
F	122	121
Hg	0.4	0.4
Mn	98.8	6.8
Mo	15.1	13.7
Ni	42.1	
Pb	69.6	25.2
Sb	2.5	1.9
Se	4.2	
Sn	9.6	
V	65.4	
Zr	145	

Table 7.2 shows some estimates for trace metals from a coal gasification process (3).

Often overlooked in project evaluation are the baseline conditions of the environment. Before process installation or use in an area, existing levels of air, water, and soil contamination must be determined for those hazardous materials that may be discharged. For pollutants that have short-term physiological effects, such as ozone for 1 hr or carbon monoxide (CO) for 1 and 8 hr (4), it is particularly important to obtain data for the worst short-term interval during the year. As an example, municipal parking garages adjacent to shopping districts are often designed on the basis of the thirtieth busiest commercial sales day of the year. Exposure of individuals with coronary heart disease to CO at levels from 37 to 63 ppm for 1.5–4 hr has resulted in statistically significant increases in anginal distress (5–7). The air standards designed to protect these and other hypersusceptible individuals call for limitations for CO of 35 ppm over 1 hr, and 9 ppm over 8 hr, to be exceeded *no more than once per year* (4). Hence, use of the process design criteria for health considerations is inadequate. Baseline information must be gathered for the highest and second highest hourly and eight-hourly average for CO before the impact of a new shopping complex can be evaluated.

Since air and water pollutants, and to a lesser extent soil contaminants, do not entirely remain where they are initially discharged, the dispersion of toxic materials must be estimated. The effects of topography and meteorology are of importance in this determination for air, and those of hydrology for water. Transport of materials in air and water to locations remote from their emissions is well documented. As examples, industrial particulate plumes have been traced for tens of kilometers from their sources (8). Elevated sulfate concentrations, measured in rural and suburban air, have been attributed to sulfur dioxide sources even more distant (9,10). Not as obvious, but of paramount importance, is the level of degradation produced, in the immediate area and remotely, in air, water, and soil by source emissions. Transport of hazardous materials may be physical, as in the case of automobiles and airplanes, as well as meteorological. A more in-depth discussion of methods to estimate pollutant dispersion appears in Chapters 8 and 9.

The evaluation of a specific energy-producing or using facility should then include consideration of most of the following categories in order to adequately characterize the discharge and spread of hazardous materials:

1. Raw materials: chemical and/or physical structure; constituents; amounts.
2. Process design: conversion conditions; product types and amounts; "trace substances"; solvents; absorbents; scrubbing liquids; catalysts; other materials in the process; material balances on major and "trace" components.
3. Process operation: start-up; shutdown; pollutant discharges during expected intermittent operation.
4. Emissions: pollution control equipment; maintenance of control devices; transfer of pollutant from one phase to another; production of undesirable by-products.
5. Interaction of site with source: meteorology; topography; hydrology; physical design of installation; transportation.

6. Interaction of source with existing sources: regional air and water considerations; existing air and water quality; nondegradation; air and water quality modeling.

REFERENCES

1. National Academy of Sciences. *Particulate Polycyclic Organic Matter*. NAS, Washington, DC, 1972.
2. United States Environmental Protection Agency. *Compilation of air pollutant emission factors* (2nd ed.) AP-42, U.S. Government Printing Office, Washington, DC, 1973.
3. Wadden, R. A. Coal hydrogenation and environmental health. *Environ. Health Perspect*. **14**:201–206, 1976.
4. United States Environmental Protection Agency. National primary and secondary ambient air quality standards. *Fed. Regist*. **36**:8186, 1971.
5. Anderson, E. W., Andelman, R. J., Strauch, J. M., Fortuin, N. J., and Knelson, J. H. Effect of low level carbon monoxide exposure on onset and duration of angina pectoris. *Ann. Intern. Med.* **79**:46–50, 1973.
6. Aronow, W. S., Harris, C. N., Isbell, M. W., Rokaw, S. N., and Imparato, D. Effects of freeway travel on angina pectoris. *Ann. Intern. Med.* **77**:669–676, 1972.
7. Aronow, W. S. and Isbell, M. W. Carbon monoxide effect on exercised-induced angina pectoris. *Ann. Intern. Med.* **79**:392–395, 1973.
8. Lyons, W. A. and Pease, S. R. Detection of particulate air pollution plumes from major point sources using ERTS-1 imagery. *Bull. Am. Meteorol. Soc.* **54**:1163–1172, 1973.
9. Altshuller, A. P. Atmospheric sulfur dioxide and sulfate: Distribution of concentration at urban and nonurban sites in the United States. *Environ. Sci. and Tech.* **7**:709–712, 1973.
10. Charlson, R. J., Vanderpol, A. H., Covert, D. S., Waggoner, A. P., and Ahlquist, N. C. Sulfuric acid-ammonium sulfate aerosol: Optical detection in the St. Louis region. *Science*. **184**:156–158, 1974.

8

DISPERSAL OF POLLUTANTS IN AIR

Lyndon R. Babcock, Robert J. Allen, Edward J. Koval, and Niren L. Nagda

Estimation of air pollution levels can be a central requirement for many environmental impact statements. A variety of dispersion models are being employed for such estimation. The purpose of this chapter is to describe and compare several of the commonly used models.

The transport of air pollutants from sources to receptors is a vital consideration because emissions might be considered of little consequence until they cause damage to human or other receptors. Under some conditions, emissions are greatly diluted in a short time; at other times, not very much diluted at all. In order to estimate whether adverse effects will occur, it is necessary to know how much of a given emission will arrive at a particular receptor point.

Knowledge of urban meteorology remains incomplete, but this does not mean that dispersion calculations should be ignored. The goal is to predict

Adapted from Lecture V of "Land-Use Aspects of Air Quality Management," a videotaped lecture series prepared by the University of Illinois for the U.S. Environmental Protection Agency (EPA), 1973.

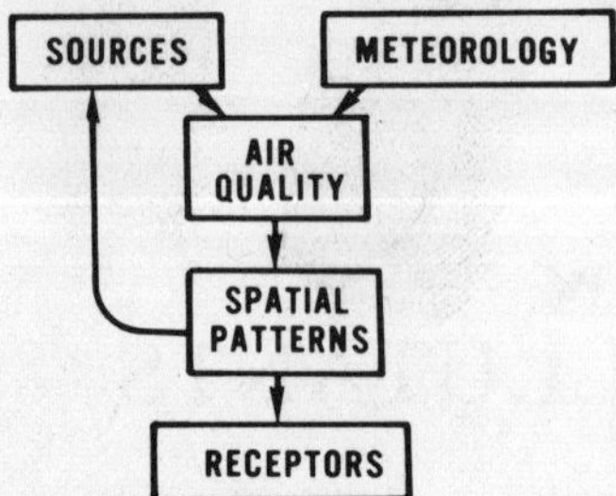

Figure 8.1. Air quality system.

how an arrangement of sources will affect the air quality at receptor locations. Whichever dispersion model is used, as Figure 8.1 indicates, it should relate the sources, meteorology, and spatial patterns to air quality experienced by receptors.

DISPERSION MODELS

In general there are three basic dispersion models: box, plume, and puff. The box model is the simplest and the puff the most complicated. These three types form the basis of almost all dispersion simulations that are in use today.

The box model is so named for obvious reasons. The region is approximated as having definite sides and a lid as well as a flat bottom at ground level, as shown on Figure 8.2. The flow of air is assumed to be in one end and out the other. The sources within the box are modeled as a completely mixed and dispersed area-wide source. The equation for this model is

$$C = q_0 + \frac{Q}{DHU} \tag{8.1}$$

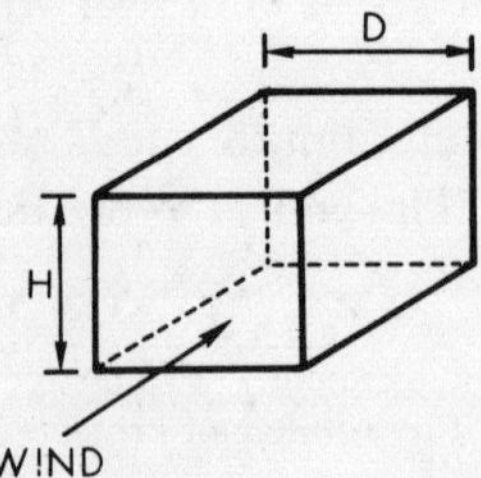

Figure 8.2. Box model.

where

C = concentration anywhere in the box
q_0 = incoming (background) pollution concentration
Q = source strength within the box, mass/time
D = width of the land area
H = mixing height
U = wind speed

Note that the length of the city has no effect on the result; the important dimensions are simply the crosswind distance D and the mixing height H.

The calculations for the box model are straightforward and useful for "back-of-the-envelope" approximations that can help define a problem. The limitations are obvious. Urban emissions from point and line sources do not get uniformly back-mixed within a clearly defined rectangular volume. At certain places within the box, the pollution level would be much higher or much lower than that calculated.

Plume models have been developed as a more realistic representation of pollutant dispersion. With realism, unfortunately, comes complexity. With a plume model it is possible to treat sources individually rather than combining them as in the box model (1,2). As a plume moves downwind it spreads vertically and horizontally as shown on Figure 8.3. The concentration varies in space. The following Gaussian equation describes a plume model that includes characterization of each source

$$C_{x,y,z} = \frac{Q}{2\pi\sigma_y\sigma_z U} \exp\left[-\frac{1}{2}\left(\frac{y}{\sigma_y}\right)^2\right]\left\{\exp\left[-\frac{1}{2}\left(\frac{z-H}{\sigma_z}\right)^2\right] + \exp\left[-\frac{1}{2}\left(\frac{z+H}{\sigma_z}\right)^2\right]\right\} \tag{8.2}$$

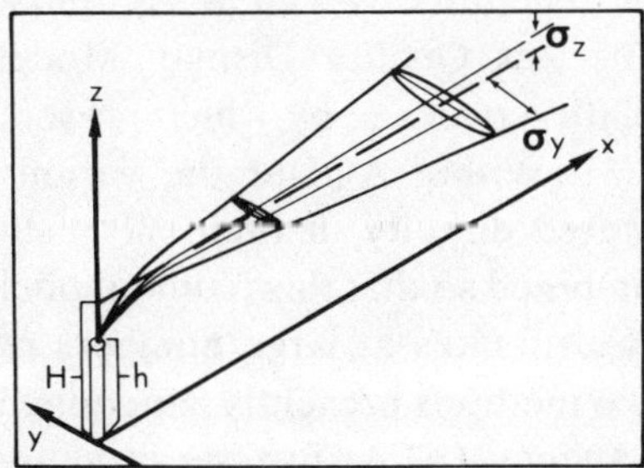

Figure 8.3. Plume dispersion.

where

C = concentration
Q = source emission rate
U = wind speed
σ_y = lateral spread of the plume (a function of downwind distance x)
σ_z = vertical spread of the plume (a function of downwind distance x)
H = effective stack height
x,y,z = coordinate position of receptor point

The total concentration at a receptor point is the sum of the contributions from all sources plus the background concentration.

The equation is obviously much more complicated than (8.1) for the box model, but it can be readily solved. The σ's are estimated from tables or graphs (2). Also note that for those sources that have stacks, the height term H is rarely the height of the stack. Plumes are usually buoyant and tend to rise considerably above the stack exit.

Despite the complexity, (8.2) still does not realistically characterize plume dispersion. Many assumptions remain. The ground surface is assumed to be smooth and flat rather than hilly or covered with buildings of various heights. The plume is assumed to be in steady state. That is, its size, shape, and orientation do not change over time. The emission level is assumed to be constant. Note that there are no time variables in (8.2).

In summary, plume equations were developed for use with single sources in uncomplicated rural areas over relatively short travel distances such as 1–2 miles. The risks are obvious when such equations are applied to large complex multiple-source urban regions where dispersion or source-receptor distances can exceed 30 miles.

In urban situations plume calculations are rarely used one at a time. Rather there are many sources and many receptors as well as continual variation in atmospheric conditions. The Air Quality Display Model (AQDM) is a widely used computer simulation package by which present or future air quality can be estimated (3). Within AQDM the various meteorological parameters are either entered directly or internally estimated. The variables are weighted and combined so that this plume-model variant yields annual ambient air quality estimates at large numbers of preselected locations. AQDM is one of two methods presently sanctioned by the U.S. Environmental Protection Agency (EPA) for use in state-prepared implementation plans for prediction of future air quality.

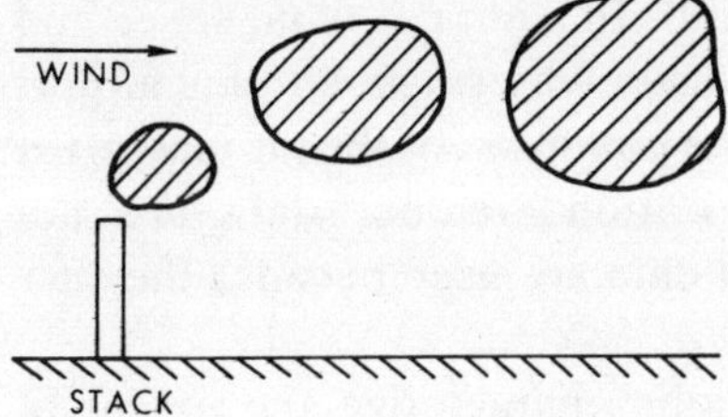

Figure 8.4. Puff model.

The final basic model type to be considered is the puff model (1,4). Here the emissions are treated as individual puffs, as shown on Figure 8.4. A similated puff can be made to respond to downwind weather changes. This model includes time variables. Otherwise application of the puff model is similar to that for the plume model. The time considerations and the differential nature of the puff equation make it difficult and expensive to apply to a complex multiple-source region, unless large-core, low-cost computer facilities are available.

METEOROLOGICAL AND DISPERSION VARIABLES

Before examining how well the models perform, it is useful to consider the model variables in more detail. The results obtained from any model, unfortunately, are completely dependent upon the quality or reality of the input data. Problems with input data are, in part, responsible for the less than satisfying performance of each of the models.

Perhaps most important is an estimate of emission levels and locations. Of course, it is unlikely that anyone knows exactly what is coming out of every stack in what quantity at each instant. Instead, crude estimates are usually made of emission rates based upon emission factors and production data (5). This approach, of course, masks all significant short-term variations in emissions. Consequently dispersion calculations often cannot realistically characterize short-term pollution situations. This is one reason why ambient air quality is often assessed on an annual basis. Where necessary, annual averages can be statistically related to short-term situations.

Emission data, for whatever time interval, must be coupled with information about the atmosphere. Weather data are usually collected at airports, which are often near the edge of urban areas. However, wind speed and direction can change as air moves from flat farm land into hotter, built-up areas (the urban heat island). In addition, wind speed and direction change with altitude, another reason why single-altitude airport values may not adequately characterize the condition of the air mass over a city (2,6). Unfortunately, multiple-location weather data are not routinely collected in most cities. Airport data are used because they are usually the only data available.

The σ's in the plume and puff equations characterize the extent of plume dispersion in the vertical (σ_z) and in the horizontal-crosswind (σ_y) directions (2). These terms are more difficult to define than wind speed and direction. Stability is a characterization of the atmosphere's resistance to change. If the atmosphere is unstable, the σ's are large and the pollutants will be diluted and dispersed quickly. If the atmosphere is stable, the σ's are small and little dispersion takes place.

Modelers have developed an indirect characterization of stability based on surface wind speed and the amount of cloud cover (2). These indirect proxies are used to define six classes of stability. After estimating the class, the σ's can be obtained from a graph, such as Figure 8.5. The method is not very satisfying; the largest source of error involves the selection of the stability class. Note the order-of-magnitude variations on the log-log plot (Figure 8.5).

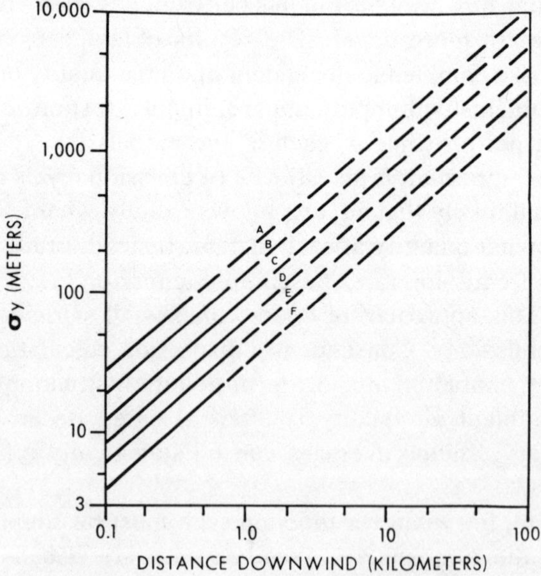

Figure 8.5. σ_y-Distance relationship.

The spreading of plumes is fairly well understood only for short travel distances—a few kilometers. For longer distances there is little experimental information. In a large urban area travel distances of 20, 50, or even 100 km are of interest. For most of the travel distance it is usually impossible to accurately characterize the plume.

Also needed in the plume equations is a value for the effective stack height of each source. Several different equations have been proposed for estimation of plume rise. The Holland equation or the Davidson-Bryant equation are examples (5). Both equations are functions of stack and atmospheric variables. However, the two equations generally will not give the same answer under the same conditions.

Mixing depth is another important variable. The mixing depth, or mixing height (terms that mean the same thing), is the height to which the pollutants can be expected to readily mix in the atmosphere. When mixing depth is low (a few hundred feet), the effect upon urban air quality can be profound. Inversions can effectively trap pollutants in a small volume near the ground. Mixing depth is the height of the invisible lid in the box model. It did not appear in the plume or puff equations, but it defines the vertical limit of the three-dimensional air space in which the equations can be applied. When temperature inversions exist, the mixing height can be clearly defined. Usually the situation is less certain.

Mixing height, like stability, is not routinely directly measured. In fact, a standard method of estimation has yet to be agreed upon for mixing height (7). Such barriers to mixing do exist, but it is difficult to be sure of the exact height or whether the barrier has holes in it. Sometimes the vertical flow of pollutants is merely slowed rather than being completely confined. Estimates of mixing depth are based upon vertical temperature soundings obtained from weather balloons. The locations where these soundings are taken are usually remote from urban areas. Such measurements do not reflect urban and other geographical abnormalities such as urban heat island or lake effects, phenomena that can dramatically influence the mixing depth.

Most variants of plume and puff models include the assumption that pollutants are reflected when they contact either the ground or mixing-lid barriers (1,2). Eventually these constraints cause the pollutant concentrations to change from the plume configuration into that of the evenly dispersed constant concentration of the box model as is illustrated on Figure 8.6.

Another complicating factor is the effect on pollutant mixing that oc-

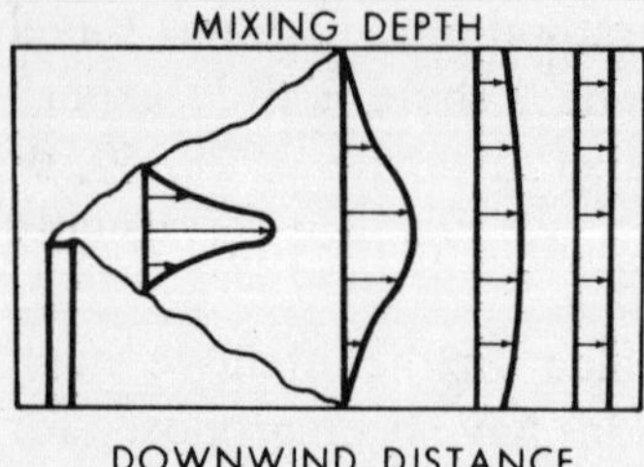

Figure 8.6. Constrained plume.

curs when emission sources are close to large bodies of water. For instance, under certain conditions Lake Michigan appears to cause recirculation of pollutants (8). In a study of this phenomenon balloons released into an onshore or lake breeze rose, went opposite to the lake breeze, then descended and returned in the onshore breeze; then they started to repeat the cycle, as indicated on Figure 8.7. This means that the pollution can be blown away only to return again, sometimes several times in the same day. The dispersion equations do not account for this occurrence. Chicago experiences such conditions to some extent on about 60% of spring and summer days. This is a significant portion of the time, even on an annual basis.

Such modeling anomalies must be investigated for regions located near large bodies of water. The seemingly straightforward dispersion equations do not take into account either the complexities of marine effects and unusual topography, or the influence of the urban heat island. Any of these can significantly affect the dispersion of urban pollutants, and atmospheric scientists have been notably unsuccessful in modeling such abnormalities.

In contrast, background pollution levels can be readily incorporated into plume calculations. The incoming air can contain pollutants gener-

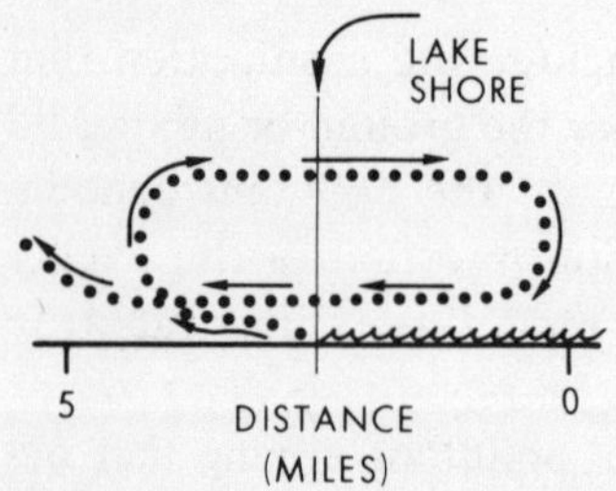

Figure 8.7. Pollutant trajectory in a lake breeze.

ated from either natural or from man-made sources outside the region. Concentrations measured at upwind regional boundaries can simply be added to the results of any dispersion calculations.

The question of pollutant decay is more complicated. The pollutants do not merely disperse; they are also removed at varying rates from the atmosphere. If decay and removal mechanisms did not exist, the earth's atmosphere would be very different than it is today. However, there is usually not enough information to address problems of reaction and decay adequately in regional air quality dispersion models. If the area being modeled is small and wind speeds are high, the pollutants are quickly blown out of the area without having had time to react or decay significantly. If, on the other hand, the area is large and wind speeds low, significant removal, decay, or alteration could occur.

Photochemistry can be an important aspect of the decay process. Photochemical oxidants (such as ozone) are simply unfortunate intermediates along the generally beneficial decay path by which nature attempts to rid the atmosphere of nitrogen oxides and reactive hydrocarbons. Sometimes maximum oxidant concentrations are found 50–100 km downwind of the precursor emission points. Because of the complex kinetics modelers usually have much less success in predicting ambient levels of these pollutants than they do for a relatively inert pollutant, such as carbon monoxide. Even for carbon monoxide, removal must take place, since no worldwide buildup is being observed despite the ever growing numbers of automobiles. Again, there are no easy answers except to be aware of some of the uncertainties involved in using models that do not include decay considerations.

Sometimes recirculation, pollutant decay, and background pollution are included by empirically calibrating a dispersion model. In this way a given set of input information can be forced to yield the observed results, even when all of the dispersion and decay mechanisms are not understood.

MODELS: APPLICATION AND VERIFICATION

Models have been used to simulate short-term (hour to hour) as well as long-term (year to year) conditions. Unfortunately more effort has been spent in developing models than in verifying them. When experimental verifications have been attempted, it is much easier and less expensive to confine the verification monitoring to a limited period (a few days or weeks). However, presently available models are probably more usefully applied to longer-term evaluations.

No one has yet attempted to maintain the extensive and intensive continuous three-dimensional monitoring really needed to evaluate the long-range reliability of urban dispersion models. A single station sampling at a single height definitely cannot do the job for the entire region, no matter how carefully its sampling probes are located. This problem of monitoring is a discipline in itself. Users should recognize the limitations and uncertainty of monitoring data. Many agencies, including the federal EPA, have discovered that they have not always been measuring what they thought they had been measuring; and sometimes the agonizing discovery is made years too late.

Application of the box model to an urban street canyon is a straightforward example of verification. The building walls clearly define the width of the box. Concentrations of carbon monoxide were measured at a mid-block location in St. Louis in 1971 (9). On Figure 8.8 the solid lines represent the measurements and the dashed line the calculated results. There is a significant variation of concentration with time. Some of the rush hour peaks are evident. For several of the peaks, the observed and calculated results coincide. However, large discrepancies are apparent. At some points the measured concentration is over three times the calculated value. There are several reasons for the relatively good agreement: the area being modeled was small; the geometry (the dimensions) of the box was defined; single continuous monitors for wind speed and carbon monoxide concentration adequately provided the input ambient data. There was no need to estimate stability and the extent of plume dispersion. Also, emissions were very accurately estimated using traffic counts that were detailed enough to indicate hour-by-hour variations.

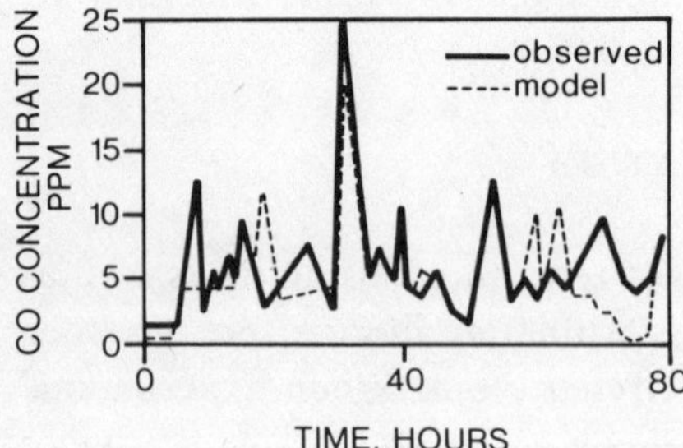

Figure 8.8. Evaluation of box model.

In another comparison box models were applied to entire urban regions for yearly time periods. For this situation

$$C = K\frac{Q}{UA} \tag{8.3}$$

where

C = concentration
Q = emission rate
U = average wind speed
A = city area
K = dimensionless proportionality constant

Note that neither the city shape, the wind direction, nor the mixing depth are included in this simple equation. Both particulates and sulfur dioxide were studied for 29 U.S. cities in which calculated results using this equation were compared with ambient annual averages (10).

Some values for K are listed in Table 8.1. For sulfur dioxide the values of K vary from 5 to 218 with an average of 50. For particulate matter, the so-called constant varies from 57 to 634 with an average of 200. These averages are for all 29 cities, not just the seven examples shown in Table 8.1.

The variation in K between cities is high. However, the standard error is only ± 50%. This is not bad for a model that almost totally ignores the urban geometry and atmospheric variables. Admittedly, this work raises

Table 8.1 Comparison of *K* Values found for Equation (8.3)

	Particulates	SO_2
Chicago	154	81
Los Angeles	205	—
Philadelphia	634	218
Pittsburg	426	117
St. Louis	122	27
Detroit	155	5
Cleveland	57	16
29-city average	200	50

questions: Why are the constants different for the two pollutants? How repeatable are the results? In other words, what happened the following year? Did cities keep the same constant? Did the overall averages change? Despite the questions and the obvious limitations, this simple approach can sometimes deliver more useful information per man hour of effort. One might expect considerable improvement when the more-sophisticated time-consuming plume and puff models are employed.

For plume model performance, short-term results also are available for St. Louis (1). In this case plume equations were used to predict the total contributions of highway and airport sources upon a single monitoring location. The pollutant is carbon monoxide, and about three days of observations in 1964 are shown in Figure 8.9. Again, some of the daily rush hours are quite apparent. Overall the model obviously does not duplicate the observed conditions. For a few short periods of time the model and observations are in close agreement. At other times the model significantly deviates from observations. The errors are larger than those for the box model, but the source-receptor geometry being considered here is much more complex than in the previous straightforward urban canyon example.

Next considered are long-term results based upon AQDM. The dispersion model employed in this computerized package is a simplified variant of the plume model (8.2). Values for mixing depth are estimated from stability information. (High stability yields low mixing depth.) Stability estimates in turn are derived from wind-speed-cloud-cover relationships.

AQDM then combines groups of short-term meteorological measurements into weighted annual averages. In all, AQDM computes concentrations for each of 480 combinations of weather conditions comprised

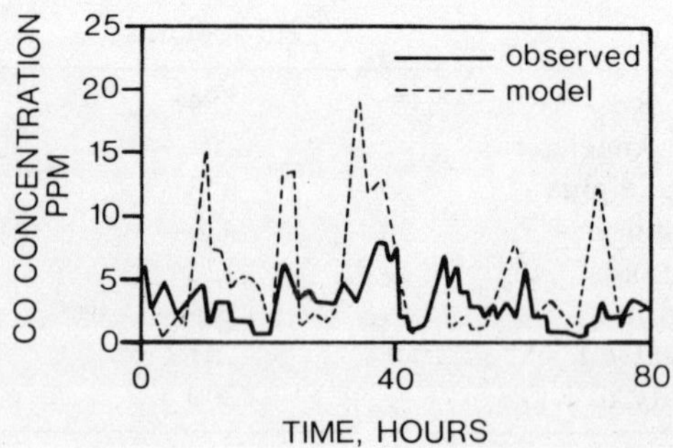

Figure 8.9. Evaluation of plume model.

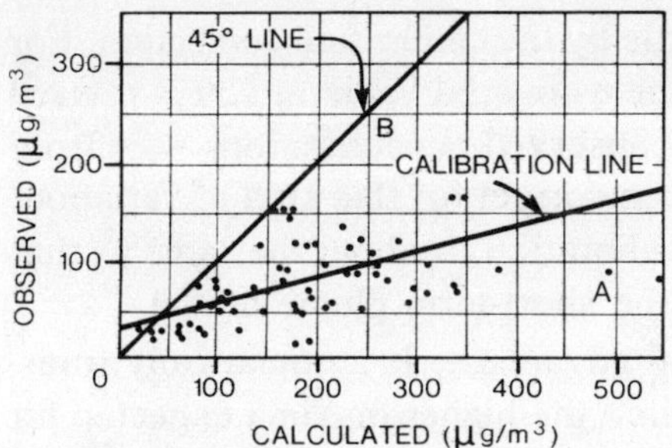

Figure 8.10. Evaluation of air quality display model.

of 16 wind directions, 6 wind-speed classes, and 5 stability classes. The annual frequency of occurrence of each combination is then determined. Finally, the mean annual concentrations are calculated as the frequency-weighted sums of concentrations for each set of conditions.

Sulfur dioxide concentrations in Chicago have been calculated using AQDM and are plotted against observed values in Figure 8.10 (11). If AQDM precisely predicted the observations, the points would lie on the 45 degree line. Very few of the points do. In the extreme, at point *A*, the model calculated a concentration of 500 for an observation of less than 100. Roughly this same sized error was noted on occasion when the standard plume model was used for a short-term comparison.

AQDM does not stop here. The next step is calibration. Ideally, a straight line or simple curve could be fitted that passed through or close to most of the data points. A linear calibration line for the Chicago data is also shown on Figure 8.10. The equation for this line is

$$\begin{matrix}\text{observed} \\ \text{concentration}\end{matrix} = 32 + 0.26\left(\begin{matrix}\text{calculated} \\ \text{concentration}\end{matrix}\right) \tag{8.4}$$

Note that 32 is the intersection with the vertical axis. This point represents the concentration in the air when emissions are zero, that is, the background concentration. It is probably to be expected that a background or incoming concentration must be added to the plume-calculation results.

Unfortunately this regression-derived calibration line, with its correction for background and other unknown contributions, still explains only 27% of the variation between the observed and calculated concentrations. In fact, some data points lie closer to the rigorous 45 degree line than to the calibration line.

Overall agreement is increased a little by the calibration correction. For example, at point *B* on Figure 8.10 the estimated value of 250 is revised downward to 100, but in this vicinity observed concentrations vary from 20 to 150. No single calibration line can correct for this kind of variation. The accuracy of AQDM, even after calibration, is about the same as that for the calibrated box model or for the short-term plume model.

AQDM does have at least one real advantage. It automatically translates annual-average concentrations into the higher maxima expected for shorter time periods. In this way it is possible to obtain an automatic indication of how annual averages relate to once-a-year maxima for 1 hr or for other short-term periods. These statistical techniques indicate that when the annual average level of a pollutant is kept below a certain level, concentrations of that pollutant for shorter periods are not likely to exceed certain higher levels. Thus, a specific low annual average concentration tends to insure that a once-a-year maximum for 1 hr or other time period is being achieved. Also note that the best data available for use in models are usually of an annual nature. Determining meteorological or emission frequency distributions on an hourly or daily basis is seldom practical. Even annual averages show dramatic variations from year to year.

The puff model represents a still higher level of sophistication than the plume model. The question is whether its use is worth the extra time-consuming complexity. The puff model simulates emitted pollutants as discrete bundles that can be made to respond to differing conditions downwind from the source. Clearly this approach is conceptually more realistic. Both the plume and the puff results are compared with observations on Figure 8.11. This comparison utilizes sulfur dioxide concentrations obtained from a Chicago monitoring station (4). The puff model

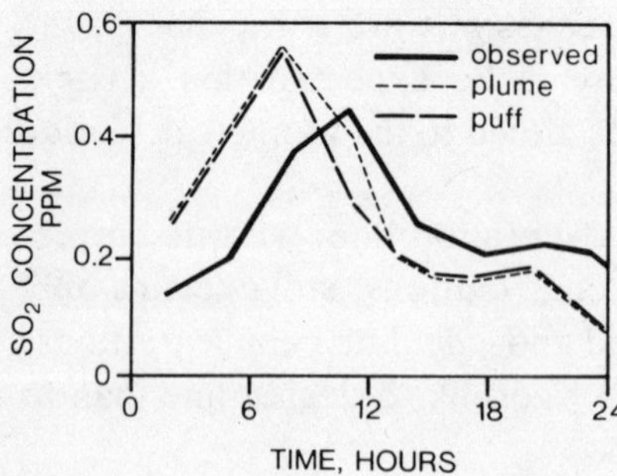

Figure 8.11. Comparison of puff and plume models.

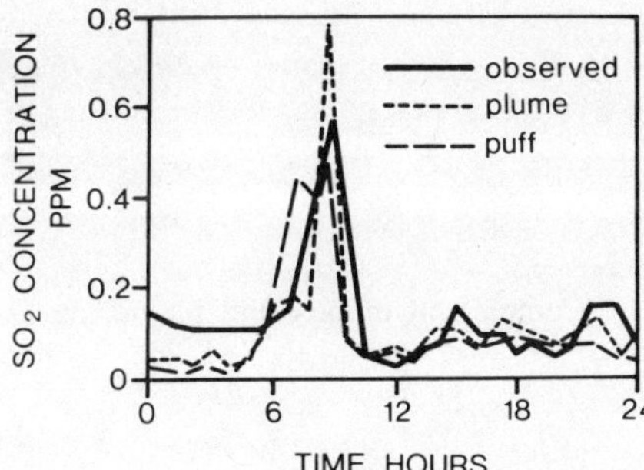

Figure 8.12. Comparison of puff and plume models.

seems to incorporate the same flaws as the plume model. The two models agree with each other better than with the observations.

A similar comparison at another Chicago monitoring station is presented on Figure 8.12 and indicates that the puff model came closest to the daily maximum, but it overestimated just previous to the maximum (4). Overall it is difficult to conclude which model comes closest to the observed results, but, based upon this limited evidence, there seems to be little real advantage of the puff model over the less complex plume model. Perhaps the situation will change when better time-dependent emission and urban-meteorology data at more locations become available. But for now there seems little justification to warrant use of the puff model. In support of this conclusion Argonne National Laboratory, developer of the puff model, presently relies almost exclusively on the AQDM alternative.

Large errors remain whichever model is used, but, in fairness to both the plume and puff models, it should be noted that the time periods used in most of the comparisons are very short. The agreement with observations seems to indicate that although there is not a complete understanding of urban air pollutant dispersion, the models generally approximate observed conditions.

If the time-consuming complexity of the puff over the plume model is difficult to justify, and if simplicity is a virtue, why not employ the box model exclusively? Clearly the box model breaks down when it comes to large-point sources. As shown on Figure 8.13, the box model gives a constant concentration everywhere, while the plume model yields a Gaussian distribution. Note that these differences would decrease as the time period increases, because during the course of a year, in most locations, wind directions would vary by 360 degrees. Likewise, wind speeds, stabilities, and mixing depths would also be expected to vary

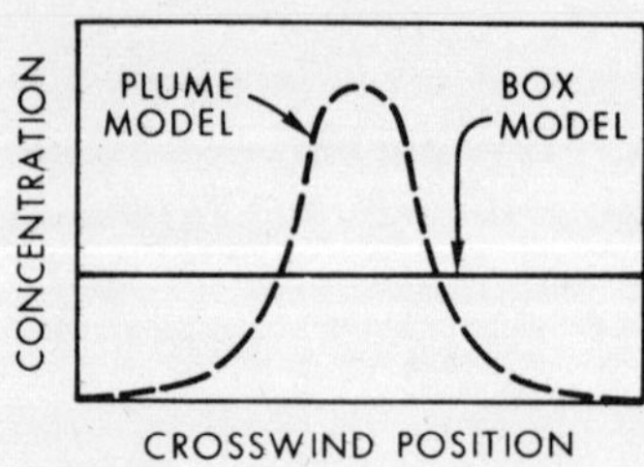

Figure 8.13. Comparison of box and plume model concentrations.

markedly when AQDM weights and sums all the 480 meteorological combinations. In some situations the results can very well resemble the crude box-model approximation.

EPA recognizes this situation. Recall that AQDM is one of two sanctioned methods for predicting future air quality. The other method, called "roll-back," is simply to assume that any reduction in emissions would be immediately reflected as a directly proportional reduction in ambient pollutant levels. Roll-back modeling neglects consideration of source-receptor geometry or urban meteorology. This conclusion can be derived from the box model (8.3) with everything held constant except C and Q. Any reduction in the emission term Q is directly reflected in the ambient concentration term C. The situation is not quite so clear-cut when incoming pollution q_0 is a sizable portion of the total (8.1).

SUMMARY

The inability to identify an always accurate model produces a significant dilemma. For example, a useful and often cost-effective way to manage air quality is to segregate sources from receptors through judicious land use control. However, this presupposes that there are presently tools to adequately define how far from, and in what direction, receptors should be located from sources. The concern is, perhaps, not so much with the models, but with the data that goes into them. In actuality, it is necessary to calibrate all the model types whether box, plume, or puff. Even with calibration there can be many weaknesses in the model. Calibration can mask errors in any of the variables discussed: the wind speeds or directions, mixing heights, stabilities, plume rise, background concentrations, recirculation, pollutant degradation, emission strengths—all in addition to any shortcomings in the models themselves.

Particularly disconcerting would be a differential error involving the consequences of different kinds of emissions. For example, in Chicago particulates emanate from large-point sources with high stacks and in much smaller amounts from individual coal-burning furnaces in apartments and commercial buildings with low stacks. Despite the much lower emission rates, AQDM studies indicated that it was the coal-burning apartments and commercial buildings that were chiefly responsible for Chicago's high ambient particulate levels. This apparent self-pollution phenomenon has led to the banning of residential-commercial coal burning in Chicago (12). The AQDM conclusions are probably correct, but a lake breeze, an urban heat island, or another effect could also influence actual pollutant dispersion. AQDM may have underestimated the contribution of the coal-burning power plants. The calibration of AQDM would simply mask such an error.

Other models are being developed. Some divide the region into many cells instead of modeling a region as a single unit. Such models should have superior performance over those now in use. However, there is still a problem with the input data. This type of model requires very detailed data for each cell including three-dimensional wind-field components. Even if such a model could exactly duplicate observed conditions, the necessary data are not routinely collected. A model such as AQDM makes use of data which are readily accessible and that have been collected on a regular basis for many years.

The most sensitive variable in plume and puff models is stability. Small changes in stability cause large changes in plume-dispersion behavior. Unfortunately this variable is the most difficult to quantify, particularly in the presence of urban anomalies. If the situation is deemed hopeless, it is necessary to revert to the roll-back method and to forget about optimizing source-receptor relationships.

Both box and plume models can be useful. When used appropriately for long-term assessment of air quality, the models can predict concentrations within a factor of 2 of actual air quality. When model results indicate that a given strategy will change air quality in excess of this amount, it is possible to proceed with some confidence.

REFERENCES

1. Stern, A. C. (Ed.). *Proceedings of Symposium on Multiple-Source Urban Diffusion Models*. Environmental Protection Agency, No. AP-86, 1970.

2. Turner, D. B. *Workbook of Atmospheric Dispersion Estimates*. National Air Pollution Control Administration No. AP-26, National Technical Information Service Publication No. PB191–582, 1970.
3. *Air Quality Display Model*, National Technical Information Service Publication No. PB189–194, Springfield, VA, 1969.
4. Rote, D. M., Gudenas, J. W., and Conley, L. A. *Studies of the Argonne Integrated-Puff Model*. Argonne National Laboratory, Publication No. ANL/ES-9, 1971.
5. Rossano, A. T. (Ed.). *Air Pollution Control Guidebook for Management*. McGraw-Hill, New York, 1969.
6. Sutton, O. G. *Micrometeorology*. McGraw Hill, New York, 1953.
7. Rote, D. M., Gudenas, J. W., and Anderson, J. *A Comparison of Two Methods for Estimating the Mixing Depths over Urban Areas*. Argonne National Laboratory, Publication No. 71-95, 1971.
8. Lyons, W. A. and Olsson, L. E. Mesoscale Air Pollution Transport in the Chicago Lake Breeze. *J. Air Pollut. Control Assoc*. **22**:876–881, 1972.
9. Dabberdt, W. F. and Ludwig, F. L. *An Urban Diffusion Model for Vehicular Pollutants*. Stanford Research Center, 2nd Urban Technology Conference, San Francisco, CA, 1972.
10. Gifford, F. A. and Hanna, S. R. Modelling Urban Air Pollution. *Atmos. Environ*. **7**:131–136, 1973.
11. Kennedy, A. A. and Cohen, A. S. *Air Pollution—Land Use Planning Project*. Phase 1—Final Report, Argonne National Laboratory, Publication No. ANL/ES-7, 1971.
12. Cohen, A. S., Fishelson, G., and Gardner, J. L. *Residential Fuel Policy and the Environment*. Ballinger Publishing, Cambridge, MA, 1974.

9

DISPERSAL OF POLLUTANTS IN WATER

Gary R. Brenniman

In discussing any water quality management problem, it is obvious that there is only a finite amount of water circulated by a water transport system. This is represented by the hydrologic cycle shown in Figure 9.1. While water is circulating through the hydrologic cycle, its quality is continually changing. Lakes, rivers, and oceans are affected by the geophysical, hydrological, and meteorological characteristics of the drainage basin. As it rains, water picks up such natural substances from the atmosphere as gases (carbon dioxide, oxygen, nitrogen), dust, microorganisms, pollen, and other airborne particles. Once the water contacts the ground it can pick up soil particles, vegetation, and additional microorganisms. Surface runoff moves to receiving waters, or can infiltrate into the ground water supply.

Beside natural changes to water as it circulates through the hydrologic cycle, there are also changes in quality from such man-made conditions as industrialization, urbanization, and agricultural practices. Although some of these conditions consume water, most of it is returned for reuse. Receiving water systems have some natural capacity to dissipate certain pollutants. However, if this natural purification capacity is

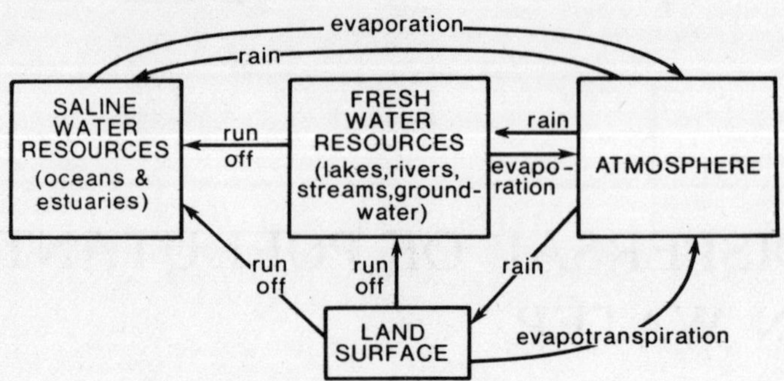

Figure 9.1. The hydrologic cycle.

exceeded, the returned wastewaters may contain concentrations of constituents that will degrade quality to a point that may prevent usage for public drinking supplies, recreation, or a variety of other applications. An example of a simple water quality management system is shown in Figure 9.2.

Mathematical models can be used to predict the dispersion and concentration of pollutants in a receiving water from various inputs. Such models can indicate if the natural purification capacity has been exceeded. Models may be employed to determine a specific water quality use by analyzing past data, assessing present conditions, and projecting future needs.

Since there are differences in the geomorphological and hydrological characteristics of the many kinds of receiving waters (e.g., streams and creeks, rivers, estuaries, lakes, and oceans), particular models are required for each of these systems. The dispersion of pollutants in rivers and small lakes and ponds is the focus of this chapter.

First of all, consider a single-system water quality model for a river or stream. A single system is defined as one where there is a direct functional relationship between a pollutant in the effluent and the concentration of that material in the stream. The pollutant can either be termed conservative or nonconservative. A conservative pollutant has no observable decay with time, nor does it disappear from the system by settling, adsorption, or any other means. Although no material is precisely conservative, total dissolved solids, chlorides, some pesticides, and heavy metals are usually considered in this category. In contrast, nonconservative pollutants, like biochemical oxygen demand (BOD) and coliform bacteria, undergo decay.

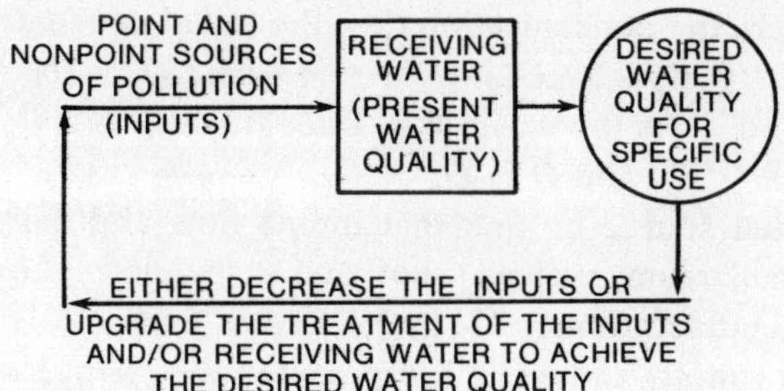

Figure 9.2. Simple water quality management system.

PLUG FLOW

Plug flow analysis is based on the concept of a mass balance for a particular pollutant around a differential volume element in the receiving water (Figure 9.3)

$$\text{mass}_{\text{in}} - \text{mass}_{\text{out}} - \text{reaction} + \sum (\text{sources}) - \sum (\text{sinks}) = \text{accumulation} \quad (9.1)$$

The change in mass is equal to the net difference between the inflow and the outflow taking into consideration the decay of nonconservative pollutants (reaction term) and the summation $\sum$ of all the sources and sinks. The plug flow concept can be applied to a river or stream using the following assumptions:

1. The pollutant is evenly distributed over the river cross section A.
2. There is no mixing of the pollutant in the axial direction X.
3. There is a single pollutant source and a single pollutant.
4. For nonconservative pollutants, first-order reaction kinetics are used, so that $\Delta C/\Delta t = -K\tilde{C}$, where K is the first-order reaction rate constant, t is time, and $\tilde{C}$ is the average pollutant concentration.

The source and sink terms may have several forms:

1. A point source will be incorporated through the boundary condition at

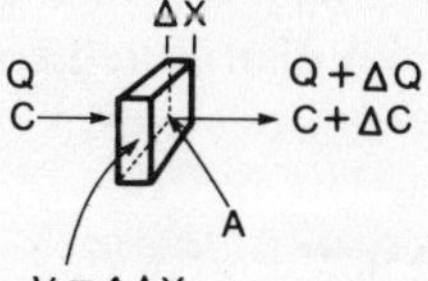

Figure 9.3. Plug flow model.

$X = 0$, where the concentration C = the initial concentration C_0. As a result, $C_0 = (Q_uC_u + Q_wC_w)/(Q_u + Q_w)$ where Q_u is the upstream river flow rate and Q_w is the waste flow rate. If $Q_wC_w >> Q_uC_u$, $C_0 = W/Q$ where W is Q_wC_w and Q is $Q_u + Q_w$.

2. A distributed source or sink that inputs flow and material along the length of the stream, such as runoff and suspended solids, will have the form, mass (added)/time = $C' (\Delta Q/\Delta X)\, \Delta X$, where C' is the concentration of the runoff, and $\Delta Q/\Delta X$ represents the change in river volume due to runoff for a particular stretch of river, ΔX.
3. A distributed source or sink along the bottom or sides of a river from a previous input, as from benthal deposits, can be represented as [mass (added or subtracted)]/time = $S_dA\, \Delta X$, where S_d is the amount of the pollutant that is added or subtracted from the river.

The differential mass balance description (9.1) can be mathematically represented as

$$QC - \left(QC + \frac{\Delta QC}{\Delta X}\Delta X\right) - K\tilde{C}A\, \Delta X + C'\frac{\Delta Q}{\Delta X}\Delta X \pm \sum S_dA\, \Delta X = A\frac{\Delta C}{\Delta t}\Delta X \quad (9.2)$$

Dividing (9.2) by ΔX, assuming that $\tilde{C} \simeq C$, and letting ΔX and $\Delta t \to 0$, gives the general plug flow differential equation for a single pollutant

$$\frac{\partial C}{\partial t} = \left(-\frac{C}{A} + \frac{C'}{A}\right)\frac{\partial Q}{\partial X} - \frac{Q}{A}\frac{\partial C}{\partial X} - KC \pm \sum S_d \quad (9.3)$$

Under steady-state conditions $\partial C/\partial t = 0$, (9.3) becomes

$$\left(-\frac{C}{A} + \frac{C'}{A}\right)\frac{dQ}{dX} - \frac{Q}{A}\frac{dC}{dX} - KC \pm \sum S_d = 0 \quad (9.4)$$

Equation (9.4) can be used for both conservative and nonconservative pollutants under steady-state conditions, recognizing that $K = 0$ for the conservative case. Equation (9.4) may be difficult to solve analytically over extended river stretches because convenient mathematical forms are not available for the term dQ/dX. Sometimes a more useful way to address the problem is to break the river up into reaches. If Q is not a function of X for a short river increment and there are no distributed sources or sinks, (9.4) becomes

$$-\frac{Q}{A}\frac{dC}{dX} - KC = 0 \quad (9.5)$$

and letting $Q/A = v$

$$\frac{dC}{dX} = -\frac{KC}{v} \tag{9.6}$$

Integration of (9.6) from $X = 0$ to $X = X'$ gives

$$C = C_0 e^{-(K/v)X'} \tag{9.7}$$

It is well to recognize that this approach cannot be applied over a very long distance in the river because K may change and the velocity may not remain constant.

If the pollutant is conservative, (9.7) simplifies to

$$C = C_0 \tag{9.8}$$

Figure 9.4 illustrates what happens to a conservative and nonconservative pollutant entering a river from three outfalls (segment A) when the river is divided into three reaches. Segment B shows the increase in the rate of flow from the input at outfalls X_1, X_2, and X_3. Segments C–E also show a decrease in the nonconservative pollutant due to dilution and decay. Segment F shows a summation on the conservative pollutant from the individual inputs at outfalls X_1, X_2, and X_3. The concentration would not fall until the flow was increased downstream from another inflow (e.g., a tributary that did not contain any amount of this pollutant). This situation is represented by a question mark. The nonconservative pollutant in segment F is also summed showing first an increase in concentration and then a decrease due to decay.

An example of the steady-state behavior of a nonconservative pollutant is the discharge of fecal coliforms into a river that undergoes a change in volume. Travel time is the amount of time it takes a pollutant to travel from one point to another in the river $t = X/v$. Referring to Figure 9.4, the following travel times and flow rates are specified: at X_1, $t = 0$, $Q = 304$ ft^3/s; from X_1 to X_2, $t = 0.273$ days, $Q = 324$ ft^3/s; from X_2 to X_3, $t = 0.213$ days, $Q = 327$ ft^3/s. The value of K is given as 1.023 day^{-1}. The concentration of fecal coliforms C can be calculated from a slightly modified version of (9.7)

$$C = C_0 e^{-(K/v)X'} = \frac{(81.7)(\text{P.E.})\, e^{-(K/v)\, X'}}{Q}$$

where P.E. = Population Equivalent (a term used to represent large numbers of bacteria), Q is in ft^3/s, and 81.7 is a conversion factor such

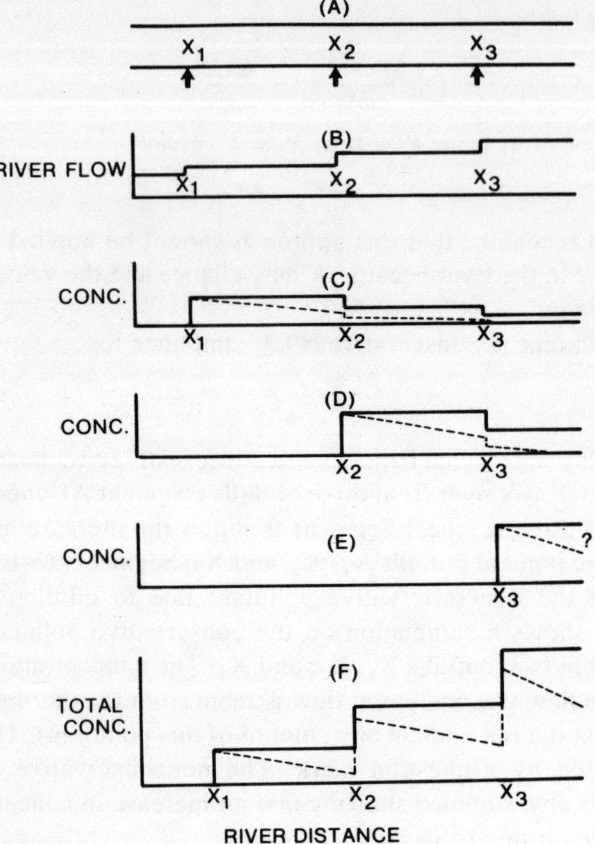

Figure 9.4. Fate of pollutants entering different reaches of a river (——— conservative pollutant; ---- nonconservative pollutant).

that C is in coliforms per ml. Compute C at outfalls X_1, X_2, and X_3, if the P.E. discharge at X_1 is 144.3, at X_2 is 432.8, and at X_3 is 11.8.

The concentration of fecal coliforms at X_1 is

$$C = \frac{(81.7)(144.3)}{(304)} e^{-(1.023)(0)}$$

$$C = 39 \text{ fecal coliforms/ml}$$

at X_2:

$$C = \frac{81.7}{324}\left(\begin{matrix}\text{Coliforms remaining from} \\ \text{discharge at } X_1\end{matrix} + \begin{matrix}\text{Coliforms discharged} \\ \text{at } X_2\end{matrix}\right)$$

$$C = \frac{81.7}{324} (144.3\ e^{-(1.023)(0.273)} + 432.8)$$

$$C = 137 \text{ fecal coliforms/ml}$$

at X_3:

$$C = \frac{81.7}{327} \left(\begin{matrix} \text{Coliforms remaining from} \\ \text{discharge at } X_1 \end{matrix} + \begin{matrix} \text{Coliforms remaining from} \\ \text{discharge at } X_2 \end{matrix} + \begin{matrix} \text{Coliforms discharged} \\ \text{at } X_3 \end{matrix} \right)$$

$$C = \frac{81.7}{327} (144.3\ e^{-(1.023)(0.486)} + 432.8\ e^{-(1.023)(0.213)} + 11.8)$$

$$C = 112 \text{ fecal coliforms/ml}$$

Note that decay of the number of fecal coliforms is a function only of travel time in the river, and not of river volume. This example illustrates the stepwise application of the relationship for a nonconservative pollutant discharged from a point source at steady-state flow for a receiving water for which the flow rate is not constant.

If S_d is included as a distributed source and Q and A are constant, (9.4) becomes

$$v \frac{dC}{dX} + KC = S_d \tag{9.9}$$

The solution to (9.9) under the condition that C (at $X = 0$) $= C_0$ is

$$C = \frac{S_d}{K} (1 - e^{-(K/v)\, X}) + C_0\, e^{-(K/v)\, X} \tag{9.10}$$

The distributed source effect is zero at the outfall and contributes to the waste concentration as the point source input moves downstream.

The general solution of (9.4) can be represented as follows (1): let $\xi = (1/A)(dQ/dX)$ and $Q/A = v$. Then (9.4) becomes

$$(-C + C')\,\xi - v \frac{dC}{dX} - KC \pm \sum S_d = 0 \tag{9.11}$$

Let

$$I(X) = \int_0^X \frac{C'\xi + \Sigma\, S_d}{v}\, e^{\Phi(X)}\, dX$$

$$\Phi(X) = \int_0^X \frac{K + \xi}{v}\, dX$$

And the solution of (9.11) is

$$C = (C_0 + I(X))\, e^{-\Phi(X)} \tag{9.12}$$

The major problem with (9.12) is that analytical relationships for ξ and $\Phi(X)$ are often difficult to integrate. As a consequence, the stepwise approach may be more useful. The use of computers in the stepwise solution reduces the laboriousness of the multiple calculations.

Beside dealing with a single-system river water quality model, conditions arise where a coupled-system model has to be employed. A coupled system refers to a stream quality parameter being forced by the output of a preceding biochemical or physical reaction. A classic example of a coupled system is the effect of biochemical oxygen demand (BOD) on dissolved oxygen (DO) concentration. Another is the discharge and dispersal of polyphosphate in a river, which forces the production of orthophosphates by the chemical process of hydrolysis.

The modeling procedure for steady-state coupled systems is identical to that for steady-state single systems. A mass balance equation is written around a volume element of the river, and all sources and sinks of the coupled system are considered. The plug flow concept is utilized again, as well as first-order reaction kinetics.

The following pair of equations represents a coupled system of BOD and DO:

$$\nu \frac{dC_{\text{BOD}}}{dX} + K_d C_{\text{BOD}} = 0 \tag{9.13}$$

$$\nu \frac{dC_{\text{DO}}}{dX} + K_a C_{\text{DO}} - K_d C_{\text{BOD}} = 0 \tag{9.14}$$

where:

C_{BOD} = the BOD concentration
C_{DO} = the dissolved oxygen concentration
K_a = the reaeration coefficient
K_d = the deoxygenation coefficient

The K_d's in (9.13) and (9.14) are not necessarily the same, but in most cases they are taken so because the data are not available to assume otherwise. For the boundary condition $C_{\text{BOD}} = C_{\text{BOD}_0}$ at $X = 0$

$$C_{\text{BOD}} = C_{\text{BOD}_0} e^{-(K_d/\nu)\, X}$$

and (9.14) becomes

$$\nu \frac{dC_{\text{DO}}}{dX} + K_a C_{\text{DO}} = K_d C_{\text{BOD}_0}\, e^{-(K_d/\nu)X}$$

Given the boundary condition $C_{\text{DO}} = C_{\text{DO}_0}$ at $X = 0$, the solution for the coupled system is

$$C_{\text{DO}_0} = \frac{K_d C_{\text{BOD}_0}}{K_a - K_d}\left[e^{-(K_d/\nu)X} - e^{-(K_a/\nu)X}\right] + C_{\text{DO}_0}\, e^{-(K_a/\nu)X} \tag{9.15}$$

CONTINUOUS FLOW STIRRED TANK REACTOR (CFSTR)

A second model employed to characterize receiving waters is the CFSTR (Figure 9.5). This type of model may be applicable to small lakes, ponds, shallow reservoirs, and sedimentation basins where the system is completely mixed. The model will not be accurate for large lakes, oceans, or estuaries.

The CFSTR mass balance for a particular pollutant can be represented as

$$Q_i C_i - Q_o C - KCV + V \sum S_k = V\frac{dC}{dt} \tag{9.16}$$

where:

Q_i (Inlet flow rate) $=$ Q_o (Outlet flow rate) $= Q$
V = Volume of receiving water (constant)
$\sum S_k$ = The summation of all sources and sinks within the CFSTR
C_i = Inlet concentration

Under steady-state conditions $V(dC/dt) = 0$. Equation (9.16) becomes

$$C = \frac{QC_i}{Q + KV} + \frac{V\sum S_k}{Q + KV} \tag{9.17}$$

If $\sum S_k = 0$, then (9.17) is

$$C = \frac{QC_i}{Q + KV} \tag{9.18}$$

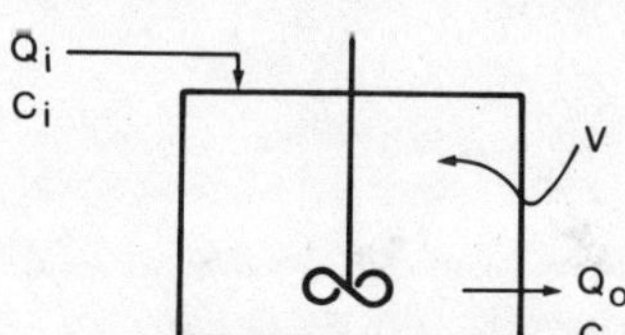

Figure 9.5. Continuous flow stirred tank reactor model.

For nonsteady state, a single pollutant system with boundary condition $C = C_0$ at $t = 0$, and C_i given, (9.16) can be integrated to

$$C = C_0 \, e^{-(Q+KV)t/V} + \frac{QC_i + V\sum S_k}{Q + KV}\left[1 - e^{-(Q+KV)t/V}\right] \tag{9.19}$$

This equation can be applied to solve the following problem.

Methoxychlor is a chlorinated pesticide that attacks the central nervous system in humans. A chemical plant is discharging 5000 lb/day of methoxychlor into a river (Q = 10 ft³/s) just before it flows into a small lake (V = 7000 acre-feet). (1) At steady state what will be the methoxychlor concentration in milligrams per liter in the lake, if it is being removed at a rate of K = 0.1 day^{-1}? (2) How long will it take for the drinking water standard of 0.1 mg/liter to be exceeded? (3) How long will it take for the lake to return to the drinking water standard of 0.1 mg/liter methoxychlor, if the discharge from the plant is completely stopped?

1. The steady-state equation (9.18) is used to solve part 1 of this problem, with the following assumptions:

$$Q_i = Q_o = Q; \qquad Q_p \text{ (plant)} << Q_i; \qquad \sum S_K = 0$$

and

$$C_i \cong \frac{Q_p C_p}{Q_i} = \frac{M_p}{Q_i}$$

where M_p is the mass of pollutant from the plant. Therefore

$$C = \frac{QC_i}{Q + KV} = \frac{M_p}{Q + KV}$$

$$C = \frac{(5000 \text{ lb/day})\,(454 \text{ g/lb})\,(10^3 \text{ mg/g})}{[(10 \text{ ft}^3\text{/s})\,(28.3 \text{ liter/ft}^3)\,(86{,}400 \text{ sec/day}) + (0.1 \text{ day}^{-1})(7000 \text{ acre-ft})(43{,}560 \text{ ft}^2\text{/acre})(28.3 \text{ liter/ft}^3)]}$$

C = 2.56 mg/liter methoxychlor in the lake under steady-state conditions

2. Equation (9.19) can be used with the following assumptions and conditions:

$$C = 0.1 \text{ mg/liter methoxychlor}$$
$$C_0 = 0$$
$$\sum S_K = 0$$

Therefore

$$C = \frac{M_p}{Q + KV}\left[1 - e^{-(Q+KV)t/V}\right]$$

From part 1 $M_p/(Q+KV)$ = 2.56 mg/l methoxychlor; solving for t

$$0.1 = (2.56)\left|1 - \exp\left\{-\left(\frac{(10)\,(86{,}400) + (0.1)\,(7000)\,(43{,}560)}{(7000)\,(43{,}560)}\right)\right\}\right|$$

t = 0.4 days for the drinking water standard of 0.1 mg/liter methoxychlor to be exceeded.

3. As in part 2, (9.19) is used, given that:

$$C = 0.1 \text{ mg/liter methoxychlor}$$
$$C_0 = 2.56 \text{ mg/liter methoxychlor}$$
$$\sum S_K = 0$$
$$C_i = 0$$

Equation (9.19) becomes:

$$C = C_0 e^{-(Q+KV/V)\,t}$$

Solving for t:

$$0.1 = (2.56) \exp\left|-\left(\frac{(10)\,(86{,}400) + (0.1)\,(7000)\,(43{,}560)}{(7000)\,(43{,}560)}\right)t\right]$$

t = 31.6 days for the lake to return to the drinking water standard of 0.1 mg/liter methoxychlor.

Models dealing with the dispersion of pollutants in ocean (2) and lake currents (3) and into tidal estuaries (1,4,5) utilizing the mass balance concept are also available. These models give concentrations of pollutants that fall somewhere between the limits of the plug flow and CFSTR models.

SUMMARY

1. Many times it is beneficial to apply both plug flow and CFSTR models to the same problem situation to see what concentration of pollutant is obtained from each model. Generally this will give the upper and lower limits of concentration.
2. Models dealing with dispersal of pollutants in water can be derived using a mass balance concept where $\text{mass}_{\text{in}} - \text{mass}_{\text{out}} - \text{reaction} \pm \Sigma$ (sources and sinks) = accumulation.
3. General solutions to the differential mass balance equation may have limited application because some of the relationships needed to solve

the equations analytically are not available. Consequently, a stepwise solution over several reaches of the receiving water may be more useful.

4. All models need to be field tested. They are only as good as the data that are being entered into them.

NOMENCLATURE

Symbol	Title	Dimensions*
A	Cross-sectional area	L^2
C	Concentration of material	M/L^3
C_{BOD}	Biochemical oxygen demand concentration	M/L^3
C_{DO}	Dissolved oxygen concentration	M/L^3
$\bar{C}$	Average plug flow concentration = $[C + (C + (\Delta C/\Delta X)\,\Delta X)]/2$	M/L^3
C'	Runoff Concentration	M/L^3
C_i	Inlet concentration for CFSTR	M/L^3
C_0	Initial concentration in CFSTR (at $t = 0$)	M/L^3
K	First-order decay coefficient	$1/T$
K_a	Reaeration coefficient	$1/T$
K_d	Deoxygenation coefficient	$1/T$
Q	Receiving water flow rate	L^3/T
S_d	Distributed source	M/L^3T
S_k	Source or sink for CFSTR	M/L^3T
t	Time	T
V	Volume of receiving water body	L^3
v	River velocity = Q/A	L/T
X	Distance in direction of flow	L
Σ	Summation of a number of terms	

* M = mass; L = length; T = time.

REFERENCES

1. Thomann, R. V. *Systems Analysis and Water Quality Management.* McGraw-Hill, New York, 1972.

2. Brooks, N. H. Diffusion of sewage in an ocean current. In E. A. Pearson (Ed.), *Proceedings of the International Conference on Waste Disposal in the Marine Environment*. Pergamon Press, New York, 1960, pp. 246–267.

3. Csanady, G. T. Dispersal of effluents in the Great Lakes. *Water Res*. **4**:79–114, 1970.

4. O'Connor, D. J. Estuarine distribution of non-conservative substances. *J. Sanit. Eng*. **91**:23–42, 1965.

5. O'Connor, D. J. Oxygen balance of an estuary. *J. Sanit. Eng*. **86**:35–55, 1960.

EVALUATION OF PLANNING ALTERNATIVES

10

POLLUTANTS WITH AND WITHOUT STANDARDS

Arthur H. Wolff and Richard A. Wadden

In recent years there has been increasing demand from scientific and public sectors to evaluate the environmental consequences of a variety of human-directed activities. Certainly many, if not most, new projects for the production, distribution, and the use of energy will significantly impact the environment and, therefore, warrant such evaluative procedures. The term commonly used to describe this type of evaluative procedure is the "environmental impact statement."

The demand for "impact statements" was an outgrowth of the "ecology" awareness of the 1960s and, in our view, has been inordinately influenced by ecologically concerned and conservation-oriented citizens and groups. As a result, impact statements were often designed principally to protect natural resources and, as suggested in a recent *Science* editorial (1), have increasingly been used to satisfy "ecofreaks." It seems that the definition of "natural resources" often excludes humans because environmental impact statements generally have ignored or given inadequate attention to the effects of environmental pollutants on human health. It is this deficiency—that is, the failure to adequately evaluate the health consequences of environmental pollutants—that is the raison d'etre of this volume.

Although the theme of this discussion specifically relates to environmental health impacts we cannot lose sight of the real world where selection of the "best" plans or alternatives will be based not solely on health considerations but rather, at least conceptually, on various cost-benefit considerations. The word "conceptually" is used advisedly because in many instances the public health risks are ill-defined or unknown, and almost always controversial. Consequently, it is usually possible to quantify or monetize the strictly economic aspects of a project with much greater precision and accuracy than can be done for any attendant health risks. Indeed in most instances it will be possible to make only very imprecise estimates of the types and magnitude of health effects that may be associated with environmental pollutants. But, as has been discussed, many suspect substances cannot be assumed to be safe just because definitive evidence or precise data regarding health effects is not yet available.

Let us now consider the factors and approaches that can be used in the evaluation of the health impacts from pollutants. When analyzing a particular project that may discharge environmental pollutants, a set of alternative plans are available for evaluation and comparison. The types of alternative plans that may be developed will depend on the nature of the particular project under consideration. For example, with a fossil-fuel burning power plant, the alternatives may include a number of geographical sites and different types of control equipment. Or, in the case of a highway network, several alternate highway routes and vehicle loadings can be compared. As previously noted, the selection of the "best" alternative will be based on a variety of cost-benefit factors but our discussion here focuses only on the public health criteria that should be considered in the evaluation and decision process.

In considering public health criteria it is convenient to classify pollutants of interest into two broad categories: (1) pollutants for which there are standards based on recognized health effects; and (2) pollutants generally considered to be toxic substances but for which no standards have yet been developed. Many projects, of course, may involve pollutants that fall into both categories.

POLLUTANTS WITH STANDARDS

For pollutants with environmental standards (e.g., sulfur dioxide and carbon monoxide in air; phenol and mercury in water) concentrations in air or water can be calculated from the predicted pollutant discharge rates and appropriate dispersion models. If the calculated environmental concentrations from a given planning alternative exceed the standard, the plan should be modified accordingly or rejected.

Even in instances where the environmental concentrations of a particular plan are below the applicable standards it will be useful to calculate the exposure levels. Subsequent estimation of health impact will enable a comparison to be made of the relative risks of the various alternatives in order to minimize exposure of hypersusceptible population subgroups.

POLLUTANTS WITHOUT STANDARDS

For pollutants with suspect toxic properties for which standards have not been developed, evaluative approaches similar to those discussed above can be employed. Estimates of environmental concentrations and human exposure models should be developed. However there are no "benchmarks," that is, environmental standards of risk esimates, against which estimated environmental concentrations can be judged to be "safe" or "acceptable." Thus, it will be necessary to exercise value judgments based on estimates of the health effects that are presumed to be associated with projected body burdens.

There are virtually thousands of inorganic and organic substances that occur as environmental pollutants and which are known to be toxic at relatively high levels of exposure in man or animals. However, we have little, if any, information on the toxicity of these substances as a result of ambient exposure levels. Nonetheless, most of these toxic agents are suspected of being causal factors for various chronic diseases including cancer.

The problem of quantitating the health risks and setting standards for such agents can be illustrated by the large group of environmental pollutants with carcinogenic properties. At the present time there are no feasible methods to determine whether there is a threshold or safe level for most carcinogenic agents. Consequently, standards for suspect carcinogens cannot be established with confidence according to scientific criteria. From the viewpoint of protecting the public, it appears reasonable to support the controversial concept that there is "no safe dose" of a carcinogen and that any level of exposure to a carcinogen should be considered toxicologically significant for man.

There is a need to develop models that conservatively estimate the cancer risk of environmental carcinogens in a way similar to that often used for ionizing radiation—a proven carcinogen at moderate exposure levels. In the case of radiation exposure, it is assumed that there is no threshold, and that there will be an excess cancer risk in an exposed population that is directly proportional to the magnitude of radiation dose received by that population. Estimates of risk at low doses are derived accordingly (2).

As safe levels of carcinogens for man cannot be established by application of present knowledge, the concept of "socially acceptable risk" is more realistic. This entails the weighing of the estimated risk of potentially hazardous substances in our environment against the societal benefits of the sources.

It is especially important that risk/benefit analyses of technological advances and new products be carried out before they are launched for public use. Particular attention should be directed to the reduction or prohibition of hazardous substances in the environment that originate from sources having the least societal benefit.

In our view, environmental pollutants suspected of a causal association with serious chronic diseases should be judged "guilty until proven innocent." The alternative is to wait many years for the evidence on potentiation of the disease, at which time remedial actions would be obsolete and worthless.

REFERENCES

1. Editorial, *Science*, **192**:509, 1976.
2. Advisory Committee on the Biological Effects of Ionizing Radiations, *The Effects on Populations of Exposure to Low Levels of Ionizing Radiations,* National Academy of Sciences, Washington, DC, 1972.

11

HIGHWAY NETWORK PLANNING

Donna O. Farley

Transportation plans are ordinarily evaluated by comparing several alternatives against a set of preestablished objectives, such as increased mobility, improved service, economic viability, and positive ecological effect. The plan that best meets the objectives is theoretically the one selected for development. The study described here was conducted to develop a methodology that could be used to quantify health impacts of alternative transportation plans, so that such impacts could become a part of the evaluation processes (1,2).

The traffic data for this analysis were developed by the Chicago Area Transportation Study (CATS). Trip generations, origins, and destinations were identified for a set of geographical zones identified by CATS. Within a highway network a series of nodes were located along roadway alignments, usually at intersections. The length of road between two nodes is called a link. Each link carries only one-way traffic, and it is paired with another parallel link carrying the traffic in the opposite lanes. For the purpose of this study each pair of links was identified as a freeway segment. Route mile length, vehicle volume, and average traffic speed were defined for each segment and were assigned to adjacent zones thereby establishing the geographical traffic data base.

Because the purpose of the methodology was to include health impacts as a part of transportation plan evaluation, it was considered essential that it be designed to utilize the geographic base and the traffic data from which the other evaluation measures were also derived. Both the geographic grid system and the format of data established by CATS strongly influenced the design of this study.

GENERAL APPROACH

The methodology compared the potential health impacts for each of the highway alternatives, expressed in terms of the amounts of pollutants emitted and the sizes of populations potentially exposed to them. Emission levels from freeways and arterial highways were calculated for a series of geographic zones within the study area, and these levels were related to the size of several hypersusceptible populations in the same zones. The emphasis was on the estimation of potential local impacts from main freeways, so the analysis was limited to corridors of land that contained freeway segments.

The total population and seven hypersusceptible populations were used to characterize those at risk to highway emissions. These groups were enumerated for each zone in the freeway corridors.

Carbon monoxide, lead, and noise were used as the three measures of pollution generated by motor vehicle traffic. Emissions were calculated for each pollutant from traffic data and were tabulated for each zone in the freeway corridors. This was done for each alternative. Dispersion modeling to estimate air quality was not performed because of inadequate background air quality data and because no information was available on the specific locations of new freeways.

Evaluation of potential health impacts was conducted on two levels of analysis. An overall evaluation compared total emission levels for the alternative highway plans and the numbers of hypersusceptible persons potentially exposed to pollutants generated. A specific zone analysis was also performed to identify high-risk zones. High-risk zones were defined as those zones that have both (1) a large incremental increase in emissions of a pollutant between alternatives and (2) a high density of the population(s) hypersusceptible to that pollutant. This analysis determined the frequency and locations where potentially significant increases in highway pollutant emissions would coincide with large concentrations of susceptible persons.

STUDY AREA—ORGANIZATION OF DATA BASE

The study area consisted of 645 miles^2 of land in northeastern Illinois. Within the study area the four plan alternatives used in the study (Figures 11.1 through 11.4) had the following freeway miles:

Alternative	Miles of Existing Roads	Miles of Proposed Roads	Total Miles
1	103	—	103
2	103	66	169
3	103	73	176
4	103	102	205

For each alternative, land corridors were delineated as the potential impact areas, using the freeway alignments as their centerlines. Corridors with a total width of 3 miles were established for proposed freeways, and 1-mile wide corridors were used for existing roads. The wider corridors used for the proposed roads reflected the uncertainty of their precise locations. Corridor boundaries were drawn to coincide with CATS zone boundaries, such that every zone falling wholly or partially within a corridor width was fully included in it. Emissions and population data were developed for these zones.

After corridor zones were established, freeway segments were assigned to the zones within the corridors. For the proposed corridors, segments were assigned to each zone across the width of the corridor where the segment was located, reasoning that its ultimate alignment might be in any one of those zones. Zones located where freeways intersected were assigned segments from both freeways, to account for the increased emissions resulting from more than one freeway. Once freeway segments were assigned to zones, their traffic data could be used to calculate freeway contributions to emission levels for the zones for pollutants being analyzed.

Transportation data were also available for arterial highways in the

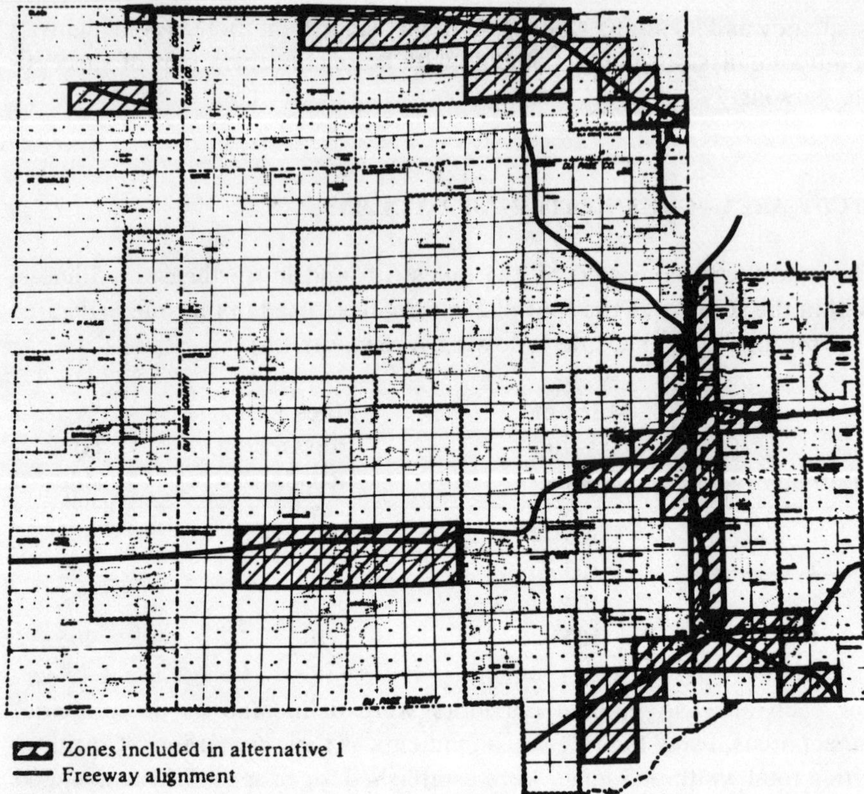

Zones included in alternative 1
Freeway alignment

Figure 11.1. Alternative 1: location of existing highways. [Reproduced from R. A. Wadden, D. O. Farley, and B. W. Carnow, *Environment & Planning,* A, Vol. 8, 3–21, by permission of the publishers, Pion Ltd., London.]

study area. Through a method similar to that described above, these data already had been developed by CATS for each zone. Emissions generated by the arterial traffic were calculated, and together with the freeway emissions they provided estimates of total highway emissions for each zone in the freeway corridors.

SELECTION OF POLLUTANTS AND EMISSION CALCULATIONS

Carbon monoxide (CO) and lead (Pb) were selected as being representative of chemical emissions from vehicular sources. They were chosen because of their obvious and documented health effects on certain popula-

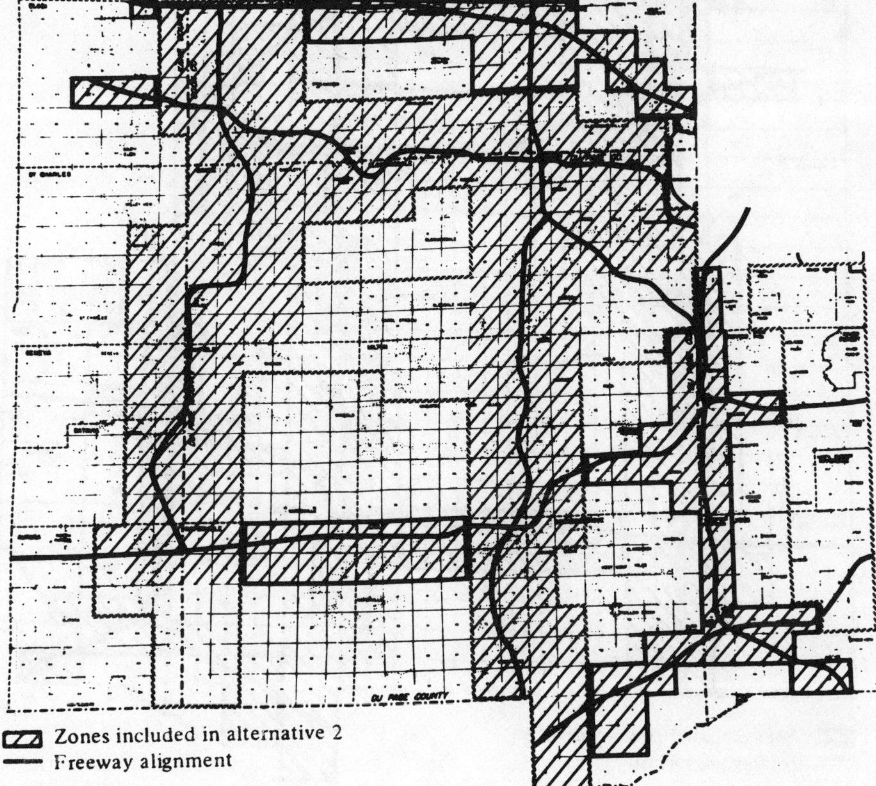

Figure 11.2. Alternative 2: location of existing and proposed highways. [Reproduced from R. A. Wadden, D. O. Farley, and B. W. Carnow, *Environment & Planning*, A, Vol. 8, 3–21, by permission of the publishers, Pion Ltd., London.]

tions and because vehicles contribute an important portion of total airborne quantities of both materials. Both CO and Pb can be quantified for this type of analysis because their emission factors are reasonably well defined, and they are essentially unreactive in the atmosphere. Each represents a different emission pattern, with Pb emitted in proportion to gasoline consumption, and CO emissions dependent on the efficiency of combustion.

CO emissions were calculated for each freeway segment and for arterial traffic in each zone by the formula

$$E_{\text{CO}} = m_v f_s \,(0.78) \tag{11.1}$$

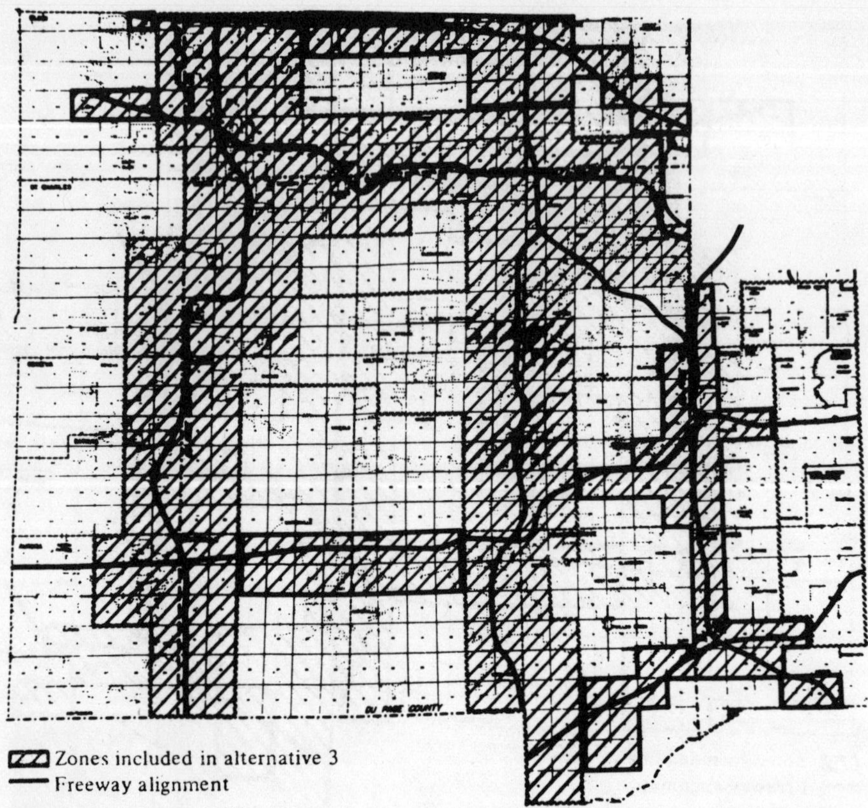

▨ Zones included in alternative 3
— Freeway alignment

Figure 11.3. Alternative 3: location of existing and proposed highways. [Reproduced from R. A. Wadden, D. O. Farley, and B. W. Carnow, *Environment & Planning*, A, Vol. 8, 3–21, by permission of the publishers, Pion Ltd., London.]

where

E_{CO} = CO emissions in gm
m_v = vehicle-miles of traffic in each segment or zone
f_s = speed adjustment factor for CO emission rates
0.78 = CO emission factor for urban traffic in gm/vehicle-mile

The emission factor was developed by CATS and was provided as part of the data obtained from them. The value of f_s was obtained from reference (3).

Lead emissions were calculated for each freeway segment and for arterial traffic in each zone by the formula

$$E_{\mathrm{Pb}} = m_v c_{\mathrm{Pb}} \left(\frac{1}{14}\right) \tag{11.2}$$

where

E_{Pb} = lead emissions in gm
m_v = vehicle-miles of traffic in each segment or zone
c_{Pb} = the lead content in gasoline in gm/gal
$1/14$ = the assigned gasoline consumption in gal/mile.

For this analysis a value of $c_{\mathrm{Pb}} = 2.24$ gm/gal was used.

Noise was selected as the third pollutant because vehicular noise is the major source of noise in most residential neighborhoods. Noise sources

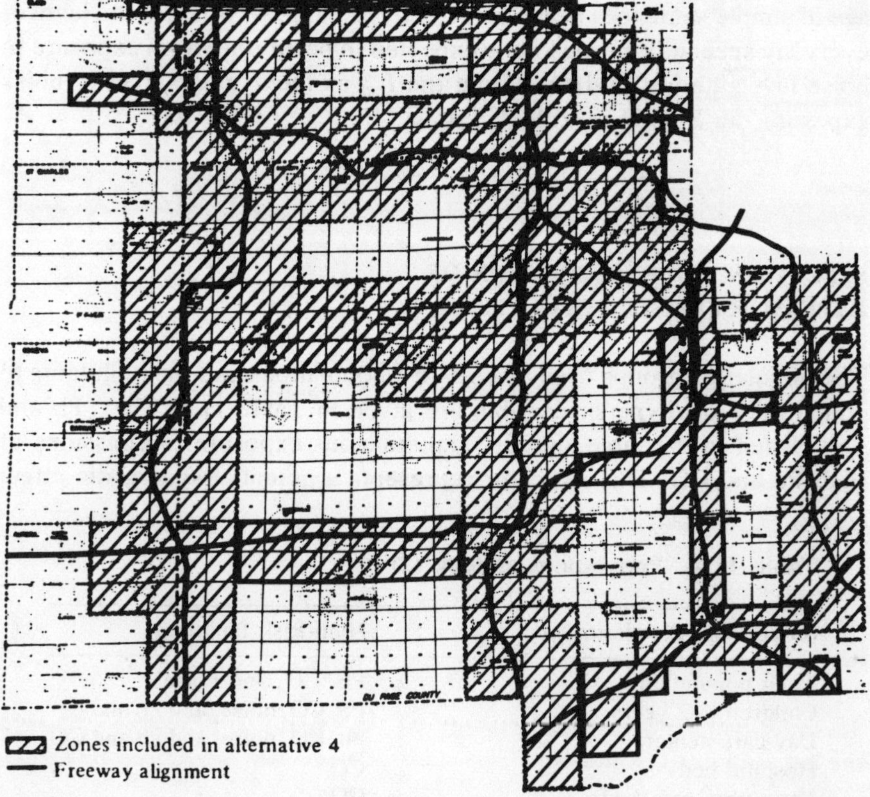

Figure 11.4. Alternative 4: location of existing and proposed highways. [Reproduced from R. A. Wadden, D. O. Farley, and B. W. Carnow, *Environment & Planning*, A, Vol. 8, 3–21, by permission of the publishers, Pion Ltd., London.]

include tires and engine operation. Its impacts differ greatly from the chemical toxicity of the first two pollutants.

Noise levels were estimated for each freeway segment using reference (4). A L_{50}, which is the noise level exceeded 50% of the time, was calculated based on estimated average hourly traffic volumes from CATS data and an assumed traffic mix of 82.1% autos and 17.9% trucks. Noise levels could not be calculated for arterial traffic because reliable average speed estimates were not available.

The freeway L_{50} noise levels were converted to an index of hearing loss called the Speech Impairment Risk (SIR) (5). The SIR is a measure of the percent of hearing impairment expected to occur in up to 10% of a population resulting from near daily doses to a given noise level over a lifetime of exposure (45 years). The measure of impairment is the percentage of simple sentences heard incorrectly at 65 dBA, which is the level of everyday speech. Hearing loss is expected to occur only from exposure to noise levels above 55 dBA. Using the L_{50} as the average level of noise exposure, an SIR_{50} was calculated as

$$SIR_{50} = 2(L_{50} - 55) \tag{11.3}$$

SELECTION AND ENUMERATION OF HYPERSUSCEPTIBLE POPULATIONS

The population groups used as high-risk populations and the pollutants to which they are hypersusceptible are given in Table 11.1. The "Pb and CO" listed in the table signifies simultaneous exposure to emissions of both Pb and CO. This indicator represents a potential synergistic effect

Table 11.1 Populations at Risk (2)

Susceptible Population	High-Risk Pollutant
Total population	Pb, CO, and noise
Children 0–2 years old	Pb, CO, noise, and Pb and CO
Day-care centers	Pb, CO, noise, and Pb and CO
Hospital beds	CO
Long-term care beds	CO
Population over 65 years old	CO
Elementary-school population	Pb, CO, and noise
People below poverty level	Pb and CO

between the two pollutants which, when both of them are present in elevated concentrations, could result in effects worse than either pollutant acting alone. Zones in which high emissions of both Pb and CO occurred together were specifically identified in the analysis.

The populations at risk were enumerated for each zone in all corridors in the study area. (See Chapter 3 for a description of the demographic and high-risk facilities methods used). The total population was available by mile section from NIPC data. Children 0–2 years old, the population over 65, and people below poverty level had to be estimated for each zone, using percentages obtained from data for census tracts located in the zones (6). A listing of day-care centers was obtained from the Illinois Department of Children and Family Services. Hospitals and long-term care facilities were taken from the Directory of Health Care Facilities, published by the Illinois Department of Public Health (7). Grade school listings were published in the Directory of Illinois Schools (8), and were checked against lists obtained from individual school districts in the study area.

EVALUATION OF THE FREEWAY PLANS

Alternative 1 consists of the existing arterial highway system and freeway network. It is used as the base case with which alternatives 2, 3, and 4 are compared. In the comparison the incremental potential health impacts are evaluated for the addition of new freeway miles and alignments as defined for each alternative.

As described above, the total population and seven other hypersusceptible groups are enumerated for each zone. Their distributions within the study area are related to each highway alternative by overlaying on these population data (by zone) the emission estimates (by zone) for that alternative. Consequently the variables influencing potential increases in exposure for those populations are the locations and intensity of traffic uses of the new freeways.

OVERALL EVALUATION

Trends in overall emission patterns and potential exposure intensities for the whole study area are quantified in the first part of the evaluation. The analysis allows a crude comparison of the overall potential incremental

Table 11.2 Enumeration of Total Population and Hypersusceptible Groups Located within Highway Corridors (2)

Population Group	Alternative 1	2	3	4
Total population	185,558	449,924	462,861	710,718
Hypersusceptibles				
Children 0–2 years old	9,638	26,570	27,271	39,840
Day-care centers	1,284	2,898	2,898	4,540
Hospital beds	776	776	776	3,129
Long-term care beds	757	1,510	1,655	2,053
People aged 65 years or older	10,488	23,463	24,494	45,109
Elementary-school enrollees	28,238	72,919	74,421	116,306
Persons below poverty level	6,480	14,465	14,890	26,154

impacts of alternatives 2, 3, and 4 as freeway plans, but does not account for the site-specific relationships (by zone) between emission levels and population groups.

The populations at risk for each alternative are given in Table 11.2. This table shows the total number of people in zones impacted by existing and new freeways for each of the alternatives. It can be seen that alternative 4,

Table 11.3 Absolute and Incremental CO and Pb Emissions for Alternatives 1 through 4 (2)

Alternative	Absolute	Incremental over Alternative 1 (%)
CO Emissions (kg/day)		
1	129,440	—
2	127,060	−2378 (−1.8%)
3	126,084	−3355 (−2.6%)
4	126,762	−2677 (−2.1%)
Pb Emissions (kg/day)		
1	3,143	—
2	3,368	225 (+7.2%)
3	3,390	247 (+7.9%)
4	3,550	407 (+13.0%)

with the greatest route miles of new freeway (102 additional miles), potentially impacts almost 200,000 additional high-risk persons and almost 600,000 additional total population over the base case (alternative 1). This is about twice the incremental impacts of alternatives 2 and 3.

Total study area emissions of CO and Pb for each alternative are given in Table 11.3. Also given are the increments in emissions of each alternative over the base case. The estimates show that an increase in emissions for Pb occurred as freeway miles increased, but did not occur for CO. Total emissions of CO stayed the same or dropped as freeway miles were added, reflecting the dependence on vehicle speed and combustion efficiency. Noise SIR_{50} impacts could not be similarly summarized since they are measures of hearing loss risk based on local sound energy rather than mass emissions.

The initial overall study area estimates were further evaluated by describing the distribution of zones and populations within the study area according to the emission levels estimated for each zone. This was done for all three pollutants, and the distributions of populations for alternatives 1 and 4 (minimum and maximum) are shown in the histograms in Figures 11.5 through 11.10. The mean CO and Pb potential emission exposures, which are population-weighted averages for all the zones included in the analysis, are also shown on the histograms.

Different patterns of potential exposure can be seen for each pollutant.

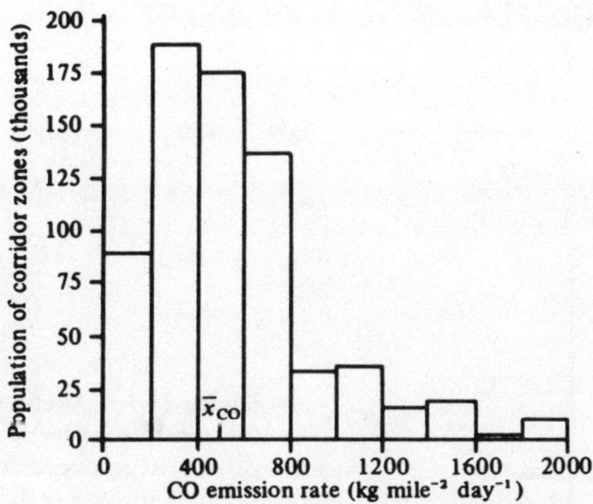

Figure 11.5. Alternative 1: CO emissions for zones in highway corridors. [Reproduced from R. A. Wadden, D. O. Farley, and B. W. Carnow, *Environment & Planning,* A, Vol. 8, 3–21, by permission of the publishers, Pion Ltd., London.]

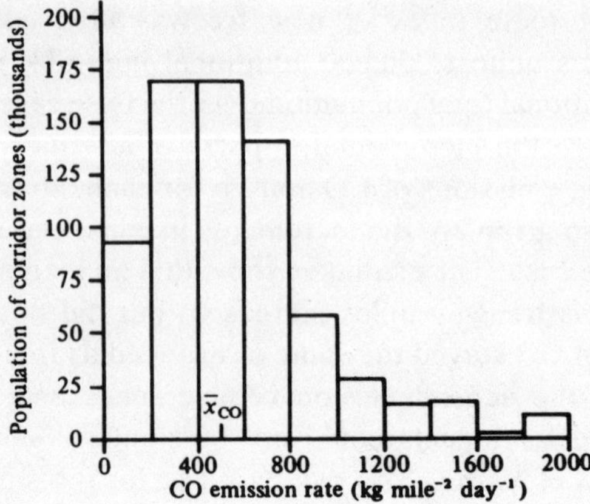

Figure 11.6. Alternative 4: CO emissions for zones in highway corridors. [Reproduced from R. A. Wadden, D. O. Farley, and B. W. Carnow, *Environment & Planning,* A, Vol. 8, 3–21, by permission of the publishers, Pion Ltd., London.]

Consistent with the total CO emissions for the overall study area, which do not increase with added freeway miles, the pattern of potential population exposure to CO emission levels also appears to be steady. In contrast, increased emissions of Pb as freeway miles increase result in a larger population experiencing higher Pb emissions as well as a reduction in population exposed to low emission levels. This pattern is reflected in the higher mean Pb exposure shown for alternative 4 and in the shape of the histogram.

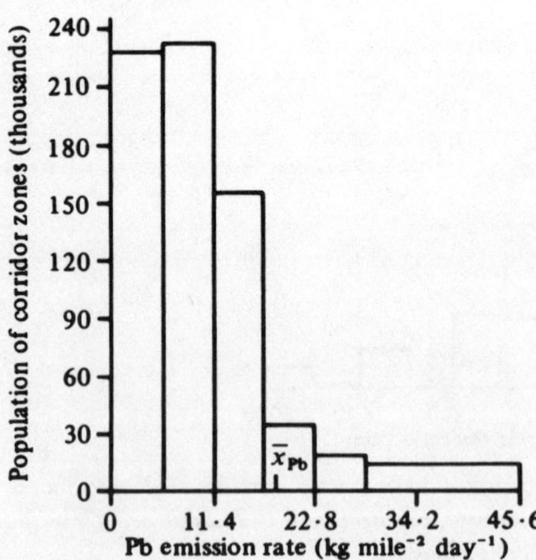

Figure 11.7. Alternative 1: Pb emissions for zones in highway corridors (2.24g Pb gal^{-1}). [Reproduced from R. A. Wadden, D. O. Farley, and B. W. Carnow, *Environment & Planning*, A, Vol. 8, 3–21, by permission of the publishers, Pion Ltd., London.]

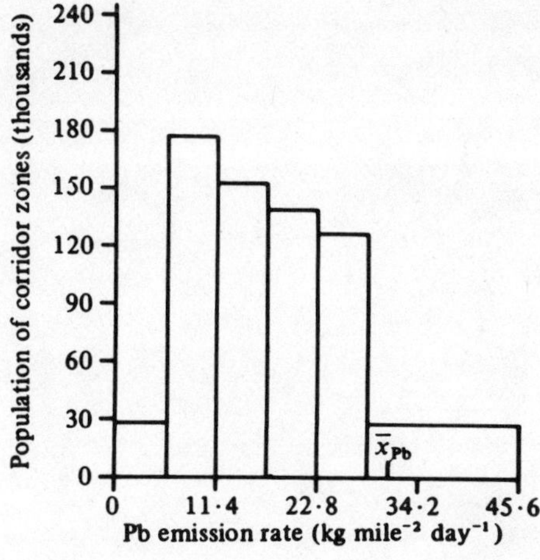

Figure 11.8. Alternative 4: Pb emissions for zones in highway corridors (2.24g Pb gal^{-1}). [Reproduced from R. A. Wadden, D. O. Farley, and B. W. Carnow, *Environment & Planning*, A, Vol. 8, 3–21, by permission of the publishers, Pion Ltd., London.]

Noise levels were only calculated for freeway traffic. Therefore the zones and population actually experiencing freeway noise impact increases with an increase in miles of freeway. The pattern of exposure, however, is found to change as freeway miles and total exposed populations increase. Comparing alternatives 1 and 4, in Figure 9 and 10, there is some increase in population at lower SIR_{50} values as well as a substantial increase at higher SIR_{50} levels. The increase at low SIR_{50} levels can be attributed to a drop in traffic and noise levels on existing freeways. The total traffic on new freeways accounts for the greater exposure at higher SIR_{50} values. The mean SIR_{50} values for the two alternatives reflect this pattern by showing similar average risks of hearing loss (from SIR_{50} of

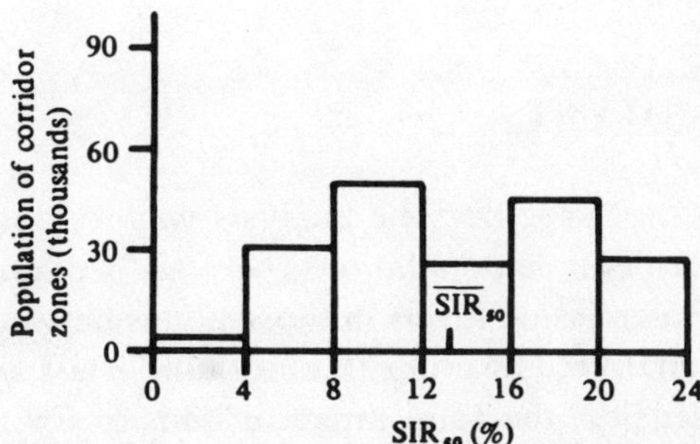

Figure 11.9. Alternative 1: speech impairment risk for population in highway corridors. [Reproduced from R. A. Wadden, D. O. Farley, and B. W. Carnow, *Environment & Planning,* A, Vol. 8, 3–21, by permission of the publishers, Pion Ltd., London.]

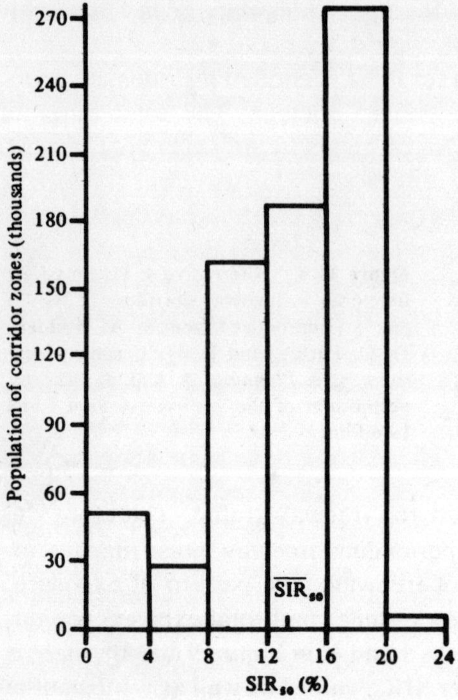

Figure 11.10. Alternative 4: speech impairment risk for population in highway corridors. [Reproduced from R. A. Wadden, D. O. Farley, and B. W. Carnow, *Environment & Planning*, A, Vol. 8, 3–21, by permission of the publishers, Pion Ltd., London.]

13.63% for alternative 1 to 13.56% for alternative 4). This indicates that more people are exposed to noise in alternative 4 and that those additionally exposed experience an average hearing loss risk similar to those exposed in alternative 1.

SPECIFIC-ZONE ANALYSIS

The basic approach of specific-zone analysis was to identify zones with high densities of susceptible populations (persons per square mile) and to compare changes in emission levels in those zones between the base case and the other alternatives. In order to determine what zones were to be considered high-density, the total range of density for each population group was identified for the zones in the study area. It was found that for most of the groups the predominant density class was the lowest quartile of their value range. High-density zones were, therefore, defined as those zones with densities that exceeded the upper boundary of the first quartile.

Emission levels of each pollutant for these identified high-density population zones were measured in a similar manner. The total range of emission densities per square mile for all zones in the study area (regardless of alternative) was divided into six classes. This was done for each of the three pollutants. Focusing only on zones identified as high-density population zones, a consistent scaling technique was developed to identify for each alternative those zones that would be expected to experience a large change in emission levels from the base case. Numbering the emission classes from 1 through 6, all high-population-density zones with emission levels increasing from the base case two or more classes to class 4 or above were designated high-incremental zones. All zones with levels decreasing two or more classes to class 3 or below were designated as low-incremental zones. When the number of zones and population size of the low-incremental zones were subtracted from those of the high-incremental zones, the difference was the net number of "high-risk" zones and the size of the population exposed in them. This incremental analysis was performed for each pollutant using the high-density zones for populations identified as hypersusceptible to that pollutant. The process was repeated for each of the three alternatives over the base case.

It was found that, as with the overall emissions, the zonal emission levels of CO remained essentially the same for all of the alternatives. The above described incremental analysis could not, therefore, be performed for CO. There were, however, 25 zones that had CO emission levels significantly higher than the bulk of the zones evaluated. They were identified as "high" CO zones, and they were used with the analysis of incremental Pb emission zones to pinpoint those zones that have both high CO and a two-class increase in Pb emissions. As discussed above, high emissions of the two pollutants is a combination for which hypersusceptible populations were identified and enumerated in the study.

Comparison of the high-risk zones and populations for each alternative, summarized in Table 11.4, will enable evaluation of the relative potential health impact of the alternative plans for those specific high-risk locations where population densities and emission increases coincide. By locating these zones on a map it can be determined where the potentially most severe impacts may occur, and adjustment of a plan may be made to reduce the risk. A map of high-density and high-risk zones for long-term care facilities is shown in Figure 11.11.

Table 11.4 Summary of Specific-Zone Analysis. All Comparisons Are with Respect to Alternative 1 (2)

		Population and number of high-risk zones					
		Alternative 2		Alternative 3		Alternative 4	
Population Group	Hazard Criterion	Population	Number of Zones	Population	Number of Zones	Population	Number of Zones
Total	incremental Pb	52,969	9	52,969	9	196,512	27
	high CO	101,421	12	101,421	12	101,421	12
	incremental Pb and high CO	8,711	1	8,711	1	74,709	9
	incremental SIR_{50}	66,775	11	66,775	11	233,497	33
Children 0–2 years old	incremental Pb	2,654	7	2,654	7	8,232	18
	high CO	5,458	11	5,458	11	5,458	11
	incremental Pb and high CO	549	1	549	1	3,646	7
	incremental SIR_{50}	3,383	11	3,383	11	10,350	25
Day-care centers	incremental Pb	611	8	611	8	1,584	23
	high CO	1,055	12	1,055	12	1,055	12
	incremental Pb and high CO	163	1	163	1	639	8
	incremental SIR_{50}	980	18	980	18	2,103	35

Hospital beds	high CO	223	1	223	1	223	1
Long-term care beds	high CO	551	3	551	3	551	3
People aged 65 years or older	high CO	7,195	9	7,195	9	7,195	9
Elementary-school population	incremental Pb	12,101	9	12,101	9	36,502	25
	high CO	16,910	10	16,910	10	16,910	10
	incremental Pb and high CO	1,840	1	1,840	1	13,464	7
	incremental SIR_{50}	15,783	10	15,783	10	40,565	29
People below poverty level	incremental Pb	645	1	645	1	4,728	5
	high CO	4,971	5	4,971	5	4,971	5
	incremental Pb and high CO	645	1	645	1	3,191	3

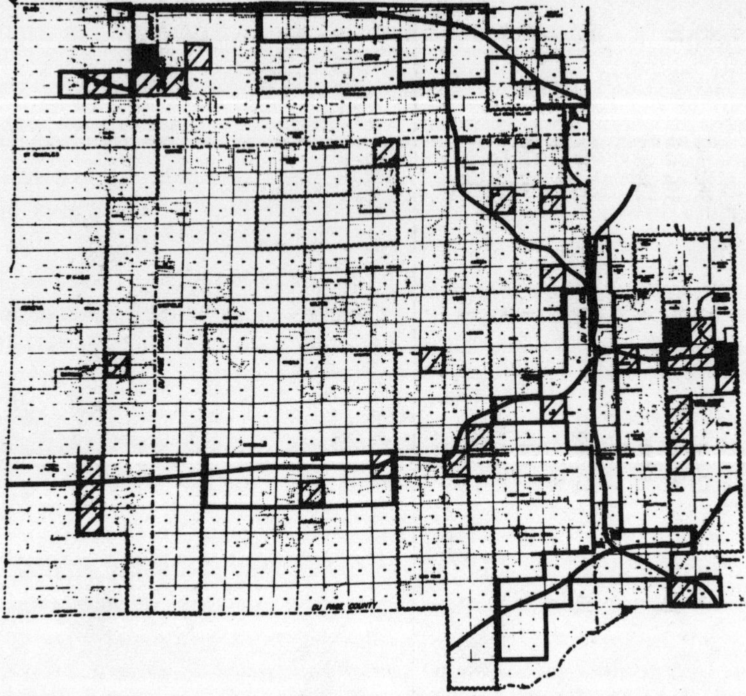

Figure 11.11. All alternatives: high-risk zones for residents of long-term care facilities in highway corridors. [Reproduced from R. A. Wadden, D. O. Farley, and B. W. Carnow, *Environment & Planning,* A, Vol. 8, 3–21, by permission of the publishers, Pion Ltd., London.]

SUMMARY

The methodology provides plan analysis on two levels. The overall evaluation describes general trends in total potential human pollutant exposure in relation to increases in freeway miles. The specific-zone analysis allows identification of those locations where concentrations of hypersusceptible populations coincide with large expected increases of the pollutants to which they are susceptible. This analysis summarizes the net high-risk zones, taking into account locations where emissions are reduced as well as those where they are increased, thus allowing comparison of the net effects of the various alternatives.

The comparison of the four alternative plans was based on the increments in potential impacts for the three "new freeway" alternatives from the base case of the existing freeway system. Because all the procedures and calculations were used consistently for all the alternatives, valid comparative conclusions as to potential exposures can be made.

The absolute sizes of potentially exposed populations, levels of exposure, and physiological response to exposure could not be obtained. If specific highway location and design details were available, appropriate meteorological diffusion models could be used to calculate air quality at specific locations adjacent to the roadways. When overlayed on population data for those locations, estimates of the numbers exposed and severity of exposure could be made. In order to estimate physiological response to that exposure, quantified dose-response relationships based on toxicological and epidemiologic studies would need to be applied to the exposure estimates.

The relationships that this methodology can provide for evaluating potential health effects of highway systems are:

1. Study area totals of people and pollutants.
2. Mapped geographical distributions of amounts of pollutants emitted.
3. Mapped distributions of densities of total and hypersusceptible populations.
4. Estimates of population-weighted average emission exposure.
5. Specific identification of high-risk zones with both high emissions and high-density populations.
6. Location of high-risk zones in relation to proposed highway alignments.

The advantage of this approach is that it compares not only patterns of emissions, but also the distribution of the people susceptible to them and the potential patterns of exposure. It can be used for any number of pollutants and susceptible populations, and as the results of this case study demonstrate, it can therefore be valuable in characterizing differing trends of potential impacts from each pollutant used in the evaluation. The method provides quantitative and graphical information on potential health impact for use in planning decisions.

REFERENCES

1. Farley, D. O. and Wadden, R. A. *An Environmental Health Evaluation of Highway Networks: A Methodological Development*. Prepared for the North-

eastern Illinois Planning Commission, Chicago, IL, 1974. (Available from National Technical Information Service, Springfield, VA, No. PB242-378/AS).

2. Wadden, R. A., Farley, D. O., and Carnow, B. W. Transportation emissions and environmental health: An evaluatory planning methodology. *Environ. Plann., A* **8**:3–21, 1976.
3. Cirillo, R. R. and Wolsko, T. D. *Handbook of Air Pollutant Emissions from Transportation Systems*. Argonne National Laboratory, Argonne, IL, 1973.
4. Nelson, K. E. *Hand Method for the Calculation of Highway Noise Levels*. Argonne National Laboratory, Argonne, IL, 1974.
5. Kryter, K. D. Impairment to hearing from exposure to noise. *J. Acoust. Soc. Am.* **53**:1211–1252, 1973.
6. U.S. Bureau of the Census. *Census of Population and Housing—1970 Census Tracts*. Publication No. PHC(1)-43. U.S. Bureau of the Census, Washington, DC, 1970.
7. Illinois Department of Public Health. *Directory of Health Care Services*. Illinois Department of Public Health, Springfield, IL, 1973.
8. Illinois Office of Superintendent of Public Instruction. *Directory of Illinois Schools*. Springfield, IL, 1971–1972.

12

ALTERNATIVE FUEL UTILIZATION

Peter A. Scheff

The recent push for the use of more coal, resulting from the "Energy Crisis" and our dependence on foreign oil, requires that we be aware of the health implications of fuel substitution. As programs are developed to meet energy supply problems, the health costs of each particular energy source must be ascertained if the options are to be rationally assessed. The example of alternative fuel utilization explores a number of health impacts that might result from substituting specific quantities of coal for oil in Chicago.

The purpose of this application is to demonstrate a methodology that can be applied to different situations and expanded as additional data are made available and to quantitate some of the health implications of switching between fossil-fuel systems. However, it should be recognized that an incomplete understanding of the effects of pollutants on high-risk populations, along with limitations in the records of occupationally related accidents and illnesses, restricts the scope of the evaluation.

The major components of the analysis are:

1. Identification and enumeration of hypersusceptible populations.

2. Application of an emission inventory and a validated air pollution dispersion model.
3. Use of dose-response relationships between environmental stress and disease rates.
4. Use of occupational accident and disease rates.
5. Application of a model for predicting the health impacts of energy consumption.

MODEL CRITERIA

1. The unit of energy used in this example is the "quad." One quad equals 10^{15} Btu of energy.
2. The analysis is limited to the fossil-fuel cycles that produce electrical power for industry, space heating, and other consumer uses.
3. The health effects considered are accidents associated with fossil-fuel cycles, morbidity due to occupational exposure, and morbidity in high-risk populations in Chicago exposed to air pollutants from fossil-fuel combustion. The effects of water pollution, and of industrial pollution sources not directly associated with the production of electricity, are neglected.
4. A diffusion model and emission inventory derived from studies carried out by the State of Illinois and Argonne National Laboratory are used to define the relationship between energy input and air quality.
5. The only air pollutants taken into account are sulfur dioxide (SO_2) and suspended sulfates. Particulates, nitrogen oxides, trace metals, and other air pollutants, and pollutant interactions, are not considered.

HEALTH-ENERGY MODEL

Figure 12.1 represents a model for predicting the health impact of energy consumption. To apply the model the relationship between energy input to the Chicago metropolitan region and air quality must be defined. This is done by first determining the total energy from fossil fuels as well as the amount from coal, oil, and natural gas. The emissions from this specific energy mix can then be estimated. Because each fossil fuel has different emission characteristics, changing the relative amounts will result in

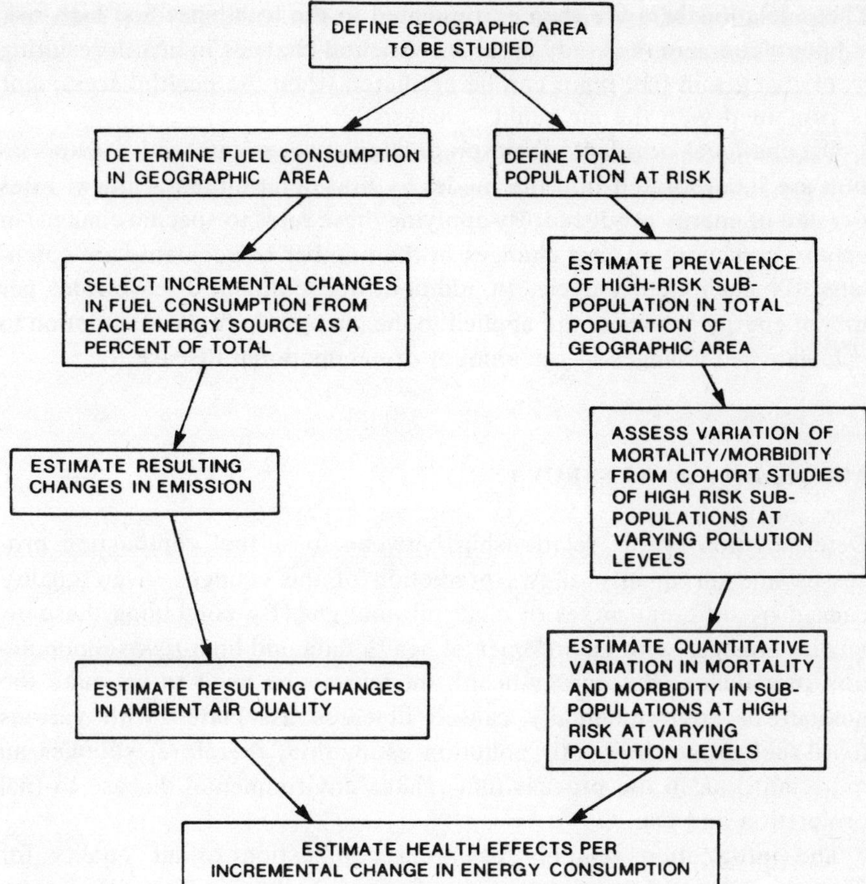

Figure 12.1. Model for quantitating and predicting health impact of fuel use.

different emission quantities. Air quality is a function of emissions. A validated air pollution model can predict changes in air quality resulting from changes in the total quantity of energy used or the fuel mix. These steps are shown in the left-hand path of Figure 12.1.

The right-hand path of the model describes relationships between air quality and human health. The total population at risk is enumerated. The high-risk subpopulations within this group are then identified and located. Epidemiologic cohort studies of these high-risk groups are used to characterize variations in morbidity and mortality as a function of air quality.

These relationships are then extrapolated to the total specified high-risk subpopulations in the study area. Incremental changes in health resulting from changes in fuel input can be predicted when the health assessment is combined with the air quality analysis.

Occupational accidents from production, processing, and transportation are incorporated into the model by first determining accident rates per unit of energy produced. By applying these rates to specific changes in energy consumption, net changes in the number of accidents are calculated for each energy cycle. In addition, occupational disease rates per unit of energy produced are applied to the changes in fuel consumption to calculate net changes in the amount of occupational disease.

AIR QUALITY AND ENERGY USE

Determination of the relationship between fossil-fuel combustion processes and air quality allows prediction of the changes in air quality caused by different mixes of coal, oil, and gas. By combining these air quality changes with environmental health data and high-risk subpopulation prevalence, the energy-health model can be used to estimate the number of environmentally caused illnesses associated with various fossil-fuel proportions. Air pollution estimation, therefore, supplies an important link in the process that relates environmental disease to fuel production and use.

The information relating fossil-fuel combustion to air quality for Chicago is derived from studies that formed the basis for the Illinois Air Emission Implementation Plan (1–5). This air quality model is used because it has been partially validated with respect to measurements in the Chicago area. Since many pollution sources outside the city limits effect Chicago's air quality, the emission inventory includes all pollution sources in the metropolitan region. Figure 12.2 shows the relationship developed between the coal, oil, and natural gas fractions of the energy mix and the resulting annual geometric mean concentration for SO_2. The basic assumptions underlying this relationship are as follows:

1. The total energy usage for the Chicago major metropolitan area, based on 1968 conditions, is estimated at 1.407 quad per year.
2. The emissions of particulate matter and SO_2 are based on the 1968 control situations in the Chicago region.

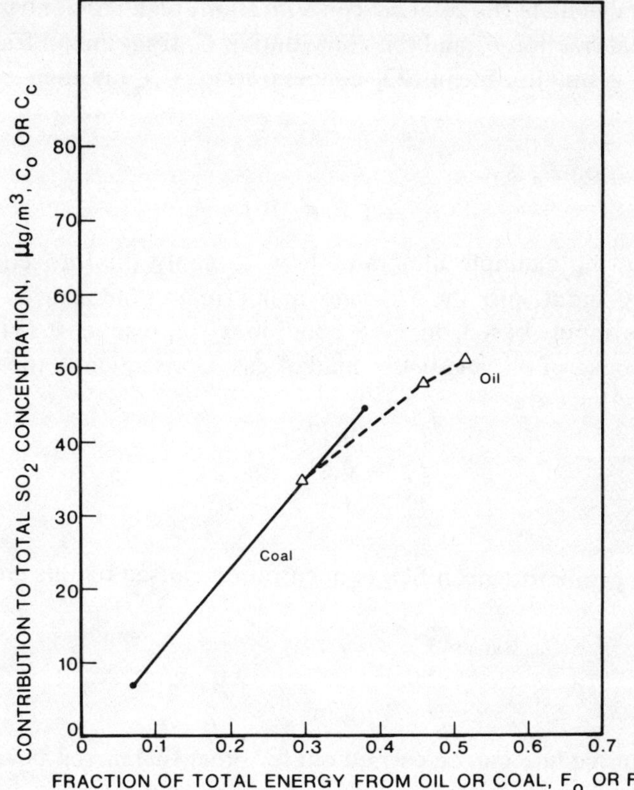

Figure 12.2. Chicago area model for SO_2: contribution to SO_2 concentrations for various oil and coal fractions.

3. The sulfur content for coal and oil is assumed to be 3% and 1.5%, respectively.
4. The heating value of coal is taken as 11,000 Btu/lb, and the heating value for oil is taken as 148,000 Btu/gal.
5. The combustion of natural gas is assumed to add only negligible amounts of particulate and SO_2 to the atmosphere.

Since calculated air concentrations vary with location, an area-weighted geometric mean for the city of Chicago is used in Figure 12.2. The geometric mean for SO_2 is then related to the amounts of coal and oil for various fuel combinations. This is done by ratioing the air quality (concentration) for SO_2 on the basis of the relative amounts of coal and oil utilized. To calculate the total air concentration, read the contribution C_c from the coal fraction F_c and the contribution C_o from the oil fraction F_o. The annual geometric mean SO_2 concentration, C_{SO_2}, is then

$$C_{SO_2} = C_o + C_c \tag{12.1}$$

The gas fraction F_g is

$$F_g = 1 - F_c - F_o \tag{12.2}$$

The following example illustrates how to apply this procedure. The total energy input into the Chicago major metropolitan area is 1.407 quads. This input, based on 1968 conditions, represents 0.234 quad of coal, 0.714 quad of oil, and 0.459 quad of gas. Consequently the coal, oil, and gas fractions are

$$\begin{aligned} F_c &= 0.17 \\ F_o &= 0.51 \\ F_g &= 1 - F_c - F_o \\ &= 0.32 \end{aligned}$$

The annual geometric mean SO_2 concentration caused by this energy mix is then

$$\begin{aligned} C_{SO_2} &= C_o + C_c \\ &= 50.4\ \mu g/m^3 + 19.0\ \mu g/m^3 \\ &= 69.4\ \mu g/m^3 \end{aligned}$$

This same procedure can be carried out for other fuel mixes as well as for other cities where a validated diffusion model exists.

ENVIRONMENTAL HEALTH AND AIR QUALITY

Identification of Hypersusceptible Populations

The purpose of this section is to propose a set of relationships between environmental quality and human health to which the predicted changes in air quality can be applied. The first step in determining these relationships is to identify specific subgroups within the general population that are at risk to the pollutants being assessed. For this example, the following three groups are used: (1) children 5 years old or under; (2) people with asthma; and (3) males age 55 and older with chronic bronchitis grades 3 and 4.

Dose-Response Relationships

Figure 4.1 showed the relationship between annual arithmetic averages of SO_2 in the air and the number of acute respiratory illnesses expected per person per year for preschool and nursery school children (6,7). Children are chosen as a susceptible group in this study because they have a much higher incidence than the population at large of acute respiratory disease, which is not biased by personal factors such as smoking. The rates of Figure 4.1 are adjusted to extend over a period of one year. Because the data were collected during the seasons with the highest illness rate, the extrapolation of the rates to one year may be somewhat of an overestimate.

Relationships between the average daily concentration of suspended sulfate and the asthma attack rate per person per day for asthmatics of all ages in New York were given in Figure 4.4. These data are applied to the present example since the environmental pollutants of New York are not too dissimilar from those of Chicago. Because of the importance of the effect of temperature on asthma attack rates, two relationships were identified. One holds when the minimum daily temperature is greater than 50°F, and the other is valid when the minimum daily temperature is between 30 and 50°F. Ambient pollution does not appear to be correlated with asthma attack rate when the minimum daily temperature is below 30°F (8).

Daily average SO_2 levels and expected number of sick-days per day exposed for males aged 55 and over with chronic bronchitis grades 3 and 4 were shown in Figure 4.2. Since this figure represents data collected from October 1 to November 30, 1967, extrapolation to an entire year may introduce some inaccuracy (9).

Enumeration of Hypersusceptible Populations

In order to apply these dose-effect relationships to the energy-health model, an estimate is needed of the number of people at risk. The number of children 5 years or younger in Chicago is 343,100 (10). The number of people with asthma at risk in Chicago P_A is (10,11)

$$\begin{aligned} P_A &= \text{(population of Chicago) (asthma prevalence rate)} \qquad (12.3) \\ &= (3{,}366{,}957)\ (0.03) \\ &= 101{,}009 \end{aligned}$$

The number of males age 55 and older with chronic bronchitis grades 3 and 4 at risk in Chicago P_B is (10,11)

$$P_B = \text{(number of males ages 55+) (bronchitis prevalence rate)} \\ \text{(bronchitis severity rate)} \tag{12.4}$$
$$= (307{,}309)(0.0285)(0.179)$$
$$= 1568$$

Note that the bronchitis and asthma estimates were made using crude rates. These could be refined by using some of the methods described in Chapter 3.

APPLICATION OF MODEL

Energy input into the Chicago metropolitan region, based on 1968 conditions, is estimated to be 1.407 quad per year. For the base case 0.234 quad are from coal at 3% sulfur, 0.714 quad from oil at 1.5% sulfur, and 0.459 quad from gas. This corresponds to 17% of the total energy from coal, 51% from oil, and 32% from gas. Applying this fuel mix to Figure 12.2 results in an annual geometric mean of 69.4 $\mu g/m^3$ SO_2. The model is then applied to three specific changes in energy consumption: Case I—change 0.1 quad from oil to coal; Case II—change 0.2 quad from oil to coal; and Case III—change 0.3 quad from oil to coal. For Case I this results in an annual geometric mean concentration of 74.1 $\mu g/m^3$ SO_2 and an incremental increase of 4.7 $\mu g/m^3$. The incremental increase for Case II is 7.1 $\mu g/m^3$ and for Case III is 9.3 $\mu g/m^3$.

Annual arithmetic means m are calculated from (12.5) using a standard deviation σ of 2.55 for SO_2 [based on 1968 Chicago air quality data (12)].

$$m = m_g \exp\,[0.5\,(\ln \sigma)^2] \tag{12.5}$$

m = arithmetic mean
m_g = geometric mean
σ = standard deviation

Annual arithmetic sulfate (SO_4) concentrations C_{SO_4} are calculated from (12.6) (13).

$$C_{SO_4} = \frac{C_{SO_2}}{(0.0475\, C_{SO_2} + 1.69)} \tag{12.6}$$

C_{SO_4} = annual arithmetic SO_4 concentration
C_{SO_2} = annual arithmetic SO_2 concentration

Geometric mean SO_4 concentrations are calculated from (12.5) with a standard deviation for SO_4 of 1.44 (14). A complete list of annual arithmetic and geometric mean SO_2 and SO_4 concentrations, along with the incremental changes between the base case and Cases I, II, and III are shown in Table 12.1.

Rates per quad for fatal and nonfatal accidents for the petroleum and coal industry and for the occupational disease, coal worker's pneumoconiosis (15), are applied to the incremental changes in energy use for the three cases. The net change in occupational accidents and disease associated with each case can then be calculated. For example, the fatal accident rate for the coal industry is 22.4 deaths/quad, and for the oil and gas industry is 2.5 deaths/quad. Case II shows that there is an increase of 0.2 quad from coal which results in an extra 4.5 accidental deaths. However, there is also a decrease of 0.2 quad from oil which results in a decrease of 0.5 accidental deaths. Thus the net change in accidental deaths due to the change of 0.2 quad from oil to coal is 4.5 − 0.5 = 4.0 added accidental deaths. Similarly, a net increase is calculated of 86 accidental injuries associated with Case II. There is also an increase of 86 cases of coal worker's pneumoconiosis associated with the increase of 0.2 quad of coal for Case II. The complete occupational results for Cases I, II, and III are presented in Table 12.2.

Air quality and environmental health data are combined to estimate the health effects of the incremental changes of fuel consumption between the base case and Cases I, II, and III. In Case III, for example, the incremental increase in the annual arithmetic mean SO_2 concentration is 14.4 $\mu g/m^3$ over the value of the base case. Figure 4.1 relates the number of illnesses expected per person per year to the annual arithmetic mean for SO_2. Applying the increase of 14.4 $\mu g/m^3$ to this relationship results in an incremental increase of 0.162 illness per person per year. This increase multiplied by the total population at risk predicts an additional 55,550 excess illnesses per year in children 5 years or younger in the city of Chicago. By applying the changes in the mean SO_2 concentration for Case I and II, annual increases are calculated of 27,800 illnesses and 42,450 illnesses, respectively.

Estimating the excess number of asthma attacks associated with an incremental increase in the ambient level of SO_2 is a more complex task. Figure 4.4 relates a daily asthma attack rate to the average daily concentration of suspended sulfates for two temperature ranges. However, the arithmetic mean sulfate data from Table 12.1 are reported in terms of

Table 12.1 Energy Use and Air Quality Summary for Chicago Example, Constant Energy Input, 1968

	Base Case	Case I	Case I – Base Case	Case II	Case II – Base Case	Case III	Case III – Base Case
Energy use (quad)							
Coal	0.234	0.334	+0.100	0.434	+ 0.200	0.534	+ 0.300
Oil	0.714	0.614	−0.100	0.514	− 0.200	0.414	− 0.300
Gas	0.459	0.459	—	0.459	—	0.459	—
Total	1.407	1.407	—	1.407	—	1.407	—
Air quality ($\mu g/m^3$)							
SO_2							
Geometric mean	69.4	74.1	+4.7	76.5	+ 7.1	78.7	+ 9.3
Arithmetic mean	107.6	114.8	+7.2	118.6	+11.0	122.0	+14.4
SO_4							
Geometric mean	14.80	15.04	+0.24	15.15	+ 0.35	15.25	+ 0.45
Arithmetic mean	15.82	16.07	+0.25	16.19	+ 0.37	16.30	+ 0.48

Table 12.2 Accident, Occupational and Environmental Disease Summary for Chicago Example, 1968

	Base Case	Case I	Case I – Base Case	Case II	Case II – Base Case	Case III	Case III – Base Case
Accidents							
Fatal coal			+ 2.25		+ 4.5		+ 6.75
Fatal oil and gas			– 0.25		– 0.50		– 0.75
Net fatal accidents			+ 2.0		+ 4.0		6.0
Nonfatal coal			+65.5		+139.0		+208.5
Nonfatal oil and gas			–26.5		– 53.0		– 79.5
Net nonfatal accidents			+39		+ 86		129
Occupational diseases							
Pneumoconiosis							
Diagnosed			+21		+ 42		+ 64
Suspected			+22		+ 44		+ 66
Total pneumoconiosis			+43		+ 86		+130
Environmental diseases							
Childhood respiratory disease	—	—	+27,800	—	+42,450	—	+55,550
Asthma attacks	7,355,600	7,375,800	+20,200	7,385,300	+29,700	7,392,800	+37,200
Days of illness for males 55+, bronchitics grade 3 and 4	84,430	84,950	+ 520	85,190	+ 760	85,440	+ 1,010

annual averages. In order to calculate the increase in the number of asthma attacks, the expected number of days/year at various sulfate concentrations must be determined. Since daily sulfate concentrations appear to be log-normally distributed over a year (14), the percent of time expected at different concentrations can be calculated. The probability that a daily pollution level (assuming the pollutant is log-normally distributed) will be less than any specified concentration is:

$$P = \int_{-\infty}^{X'} (2\pi)^{-1/2} \exp(-0.5 X^2)\, dX \qquad (12.7)$$

where

P = probability that a particular daily pollution level is $\leq C'$
X = $\ln (C/m_g)/\ln \sigma$
C = concentration
C' = specified concentration
X' = value of X at concentration C'

The probability that the mean daily pollution level will be within a specific concentration range C_1 to C_2 equals the difference between the probability that the daily pollution level will be below C_2 and the probability that the daily pollution level will be below C_1. Using (12.7), the probability of the daily mean SO_4 concentration falling within the following ranges can be calculated for each annual geometric mean concentration listed in Table 12.1: 0–7.3 $\mu g/m^3$, 7.3–10, 10–11.9, 11.9–15, 15–20, 20–25, 25–30, 30–35, and >35 $\mu g/m^3$.

In order to translate this information into the number of days expected for each concentration range for each of the two curves in Figure 4.4, the number of days during which each relationship applies must be determined. Meteorological data for Chicago for 1968 indicate 147 days where the minimum daily temperature t_{min} was $\geq$ 50°F and 126 days where t_{min} was between 30 and 50°F. The sulfate concentration is assumed to be log-normally distributed for both temperature ranges. The number of days expected at each sulfate concentration is calculated by multiplying the probability for each concentration by the number of days at each temperature level. The number of attacks expected for each concentration range for both curves are summed together to get the total number of asthma attacks expected per year for the annual geometric mean SO_4 concentration for each case:

$$A = P_A \left[\sum_{i=0} (D_{i>50})(R_{i>50}) + \sum_{i=0} (D_{i>30})(R_{i>30}) \right] \qquad (12.8)$$

where

A = number of asthma attacks per year
P_A = number of asthmatics in Chicago
$D_{i>50}$ = number of days at concentration i for $t_{min} > 50°F$
$R_{i>50}$ = asthma attack rate per person-day for $t_{min} > 50°F$ at concentration i
$D_{i>30}$ = number of days at concentration i for $30°F < t_{min} < 50°F$
$R_{i>30}$ = asthma attack rate per person-day for $30°F < t_{min} < 50°F$ at concentration i

This procedure estimates that the base case annual geometric mean sulfate concentration of 14.8 $\mu g/m^3$ is accompanied by 7,355,600 asthma attacks, Case I by 7,375,800 attacks, Case II by 7,385,300 attacks, and Case III by 7,392,800. Subtracting the base case from Case I results in an incremental increase of 20,200 asthma attacks associated with the transfer of 0.1 quad from oil to coal (Case I). For Case II the increase is 29,700, and 37,200 attacks would be predicted for Case III (see Table 12.2).

Estimation of the frequency of sick-days for male bronchitics is very similar to the procedure used for asthma. The SO_2 concentrations in Figure 4.2 are daily averages rather than annual averages. As with the asthma example, the number of days expected at nine concentration ranges is estimated for the four cases. The total number of sick-days expected per year for each case is

$$S = P_B \sum_{i=0} (D_i)(R_i) \tag{12.9}$$

where

S = number of sick days per year
P_B = number of male bronchitics age 55+ with severity grades 3 and 4 in Chicago
D_i = number of days at concentration i
R_i = rate of sick days per person-day exposed at concentration i

Summations are listed in Table 12.2. Differences are calculated to determine the incremental increase in the number of sick-days expected with each case. The model predicts 520 excess sick-days associated with Case I, 760 with Case II, and 1,010 with Case III.

SUMMARY

Most of the environmental measurements and calculations used in this example are based on 1968 conditions. The health data defining childhood disease and asthma attack rates were collected in the early 1970s, and the bronchitis data is from the late 1960s. Consequently the specific disease estimates of Table 12.2 must be interpreted carefully, because environmental conditions have changed. However, this analysis is based on observed data and quantifies a real risk if fuel switches similar to those assumed in this example were to be enacted today without adequate controls. As new occupational and environmental health information becomes available, as well as improved environmental quality data, they can easily be incorporated into an updated evaluation (15).

REFERENCES

1. Argonne National Laboratory. *Evaluation of Emission Control Strategies for Sulfur Dioxide and Particulates in the Chicago Metropolitan Air Quality Control Region*. IIPP-2, Argonne, IL, December 1970.
2. Argonne National Laboratory. *Evaluation of Emission Control Strategies with Emphasis on Residential/Commercial Space Heating for SO_2 and Particulates in the Chicago Metropolitan Air Quality Control Region*. IIPP-4, Argonne, IL, March 1971.
3. Argonne National Laboratory. *Growth Analysis Report for the Illinois Implementation Planning Program*. IIPP-7, Argonne, IL, February 1972.
4. U.S. Environmental Protection Agency. *Compilation of Air Pollutant Emission Factors*. Publication No. AP-42, U.S. Government Printing Office, Washington, DC, 1972.
5. Illinois Environmental Protection Agency. *Illinois Implementation Plan for Attainment of National Ambient Air Quality Standards*. Springfield, IL, 1972.
6. Finklea, J. R., French, J. G., Lowrimore, G. R., Goldberg, J., Shy, C. M., and Nelson, W. C. Prospective surveys of acute respiratory disease in volunteer families: Chicago nursing school study, 1969–1970. In *Health Consequences of Sulfur Oxides: A Report from CHESS, 1970–1971*. U.S. EPA Office of Research and Development, EPA-650/1-74-004, U.S. Government Printing Office, Washington, DC, May 1974, pp. 4-37–4-55.
7. Love, J. G., Cohen, A. A., Finklea, J. F., French, J. G., Lowrimore, G. R., Nelson, W. C., and Ramsey, P. B. Prospective surveys of acute respiratory disease in volunteer families: 1970–1971 New York studies. In *Health Consequences of Sulfur Oxides: A Report from CHESS, 1970–1971*. U.S. EPA Office of Research and Development, EPA-650/1-74-004, U.S. Government Printing Office, Washington, DC, May 1974, pp. 5-49–5-69.

8. Finklea, J. F., Farmer, J. H., Love, G. J., Calafiore, D. C., and Sovocool, G. W. Aggravation of asthma by air pollutants: 1970–1971 New York studies. In *Health Consequences of Sulfur Oxides: A Report from CHESS, 1970–1971*. U.S. EPA Office of Research and Development, EPA-650/1-74-004, U.S. Government Printing Office, Washington, DC, May 1974, pp. 5-71–5-84.

9. Carnow, B. W., Lepper, M. H., Shekelle, R. B., and Stamler, J. Chicago air pollution study: SO_2 levels and acute illness in patients with chronic bronchopulmonary disease. *Arch. Environ. Health* **18**:768–776, 1969.

10. U.S. Bureau of the Census. *1970 Census of Population of U.S.* U.S. Government Printing Office, Washington, DC 1973.

11. Wilder, C. S. *Prevalence of Selected Chronic Respiratory Conditions, United States, 1970*. Vital and Health Statistics, Series 10, No. 84, National Center for Health Statistics, U.S. Government Printing Office, Washington, DC, 1973.

12. U.S. Environmental Protection Agency. *Air Quality Data for 1968 from the National Air Surveillance Networks*. Publication No. APTD-0978, Environmental Protection Agency, Washington, DC, August 1972, p. 190.

13. Altshuller, A. P. Atmospheric sulfur dioxide and sulfate: Distribution of concentration at urban and nonurban sites in United States. *Environ. Sci. Technol.* **7**:709–712, 1973.

14. City of Chicago Department of Environmental Control. *Sulfate Data for 1968*. Chicago, IL, August 1, 1974.

15. Carnow, B. W., Wadden, R. A., Scheff, P. A., and Musselman, R. P. *Health Effects of Fossil Fuel Combustion: A Quantitative Approach*. American Public Health Association, Washington, DC, 1974, pp. 1–45.

13

SHOPPING CENTER ANALYSIS

Richard G. Hankett

Many commonplace activities of urban life produce concomitant effects that impact public health. Although an individual shopping trip may seem a relatively innocuous activity, many such trips to a central location, such as a regional shopping center, can have significant effect upon local air quality. In particular, the additional traffic increases the emission of pollutants such as carbon monoxide (CO), lead (Pb), particulate matter (PM), and particulate sulfates (SO_4). Each of these is potentially hazardous to human health.

Vehicular traffic patterns are characterized by diurnal and seasonal volume variations. Local meteorological conditions also vary so that pollutants are either trapped or dispersed by the atmosphere. The simultaneous occurrence of high-traffic volumes, such as during holiday periods, and adverse meteorology, such as inversions, is not uncommon. As a result air pollutants accumulate in short-term cyclic or episodal patterns. Of special concern in this regard are hypersusceptible groups such as the elderly, the very young, and persons with lung and heart diseases. Such individuals may suffer adverse effects from even short-term exposures to high levels of contamination. Thus, in the consideration of any activity that involves significant increases in automobile traffic, it is essential to evaluate the potential effects of short-term variation in air quality upon hypersusceptibles.

In the case study under discussion (1), it was proposed to construct a regional shopping center in the central business district (CBD) of a metropolitan area suburb. The center would incorporate a 2000-car parking garage and be served by an existing arterial street network and rapid transit system. Detailed traffic network assignments are available based upon "design day" trip volumes and modal splits. Since the CBD is surrounded by a mixture of residential, institutional, and community service land uses, a detailed evaluation of potential air quality effects is desired. Baseline air quality data are not available. Figures 13.1 and 13.2 show the street network of the suburban CBD before and after implementation of the proposed shopping center. Design traffic volumes are also indicated.

The task of evaluating the air quality effects and potential health risks of the proposed undertaking is approached as a 4-step process:

1. Identify and quantify pollutant emission sources.
2. Analyze changes in ambient air quality.

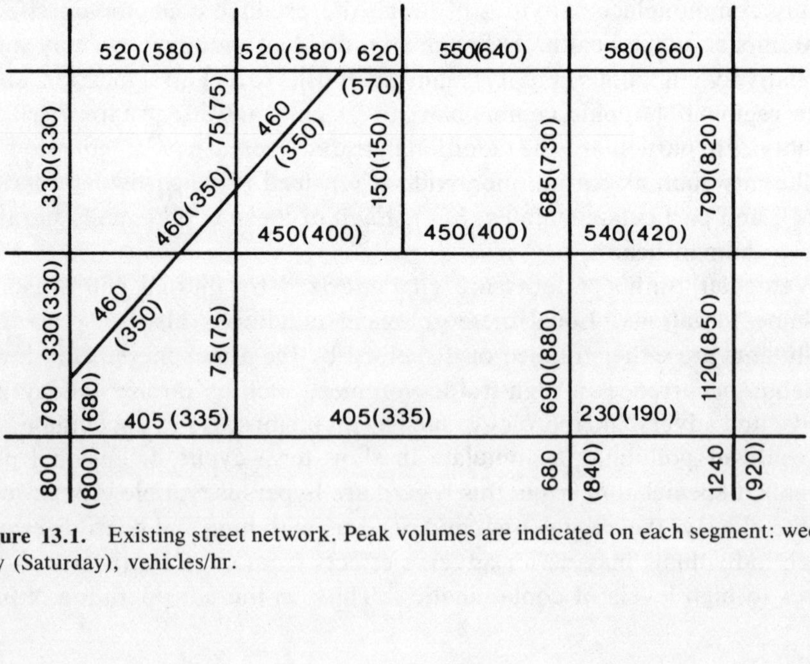

Figure 13.1. Existing street network. Peak volumes are indicated on each segment: weekday (Saturday), vehicles/hr.

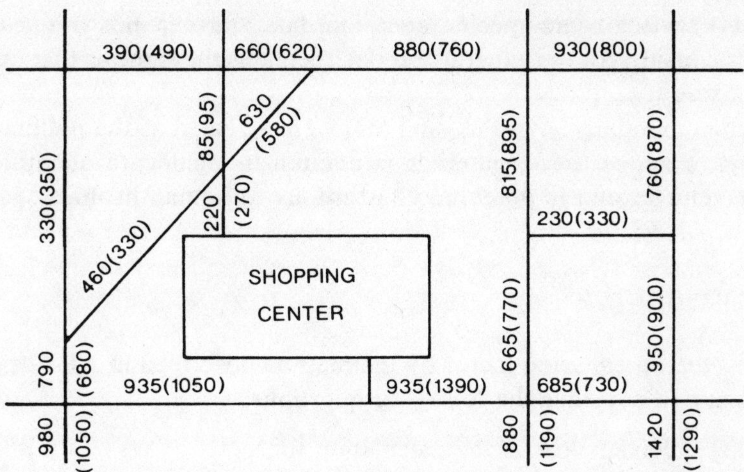

Figure 13.2. Street network with proposed shopping center. Peak hour traffic volumes are indicated on each segment: weekday (Saturday), vehicles/hr.

3. Identify hypersusceptible receptor groups exposed to increased contamination.
4. Evaluate severity of health-based impacts upon receptors.

AIR POLLUTANT EMISSION SOURCES

The primary air pollutant emission source associated with the shopping center is automobile traffic over the roadway network serving the center. Air pollutant emissions produced by a vehicular transportation facility or network are a function of the vehicle population, average speeds, idling times, operating characteristics, and travel patterns. The factors of vehicle population, speed, idling, and operating mode may be accounted for via a composite emission factor for the pollutant of interest. Travel patterns may be represented in terms of vehicle miles traveled (VMT) over a given highway network or within a given area. For the purposes of this study, the composite emission factor calculation methods presented in Supplement 5 (December 1975) to U.S. Environmental Protection Agency Publication AP-42 were utilized (2,3). The U.S. EPA recently (June 1977) promulgated an interim procedure for mobile source emission factor calculation (4) which updates Supplement 5 to AP-42. While reference (4) revises some specific emission data and expands the scope of factors considered, the general approach remains the same as that utilized in this study.

Carbon monoxide, Pb, PM, and SO_4 were selected as the pollutants of interest. Each of these materials is emitted in significant quantities by motor vehicles and is potentially hazardous to human health.

EMISSION FACTORS

To develop an emission factor by the method described in AP-42 (3) it is necessary to consider the following questions:

1. What calendar year is the calculation for?
2. What is the average speed for the area of concern?
3. What is the vehicle mix in terms of types, age, and annual travel?
4. What is the ambient temperature?
5. What is the hot start/cold start operational ratio?

In this case study, the appropriate responses were:

1. The estimated year of project completion was 1978 and was, therefore, used for both the proposed and "do-nothing" cases.
2. Traffic on the CBD arterial streets was estimated to travel at an average speed of 15 mph.
3. The vehicle age and mileage mix used is shown in Table 13.1. A population of 100% light-duty vehicles (autos) is assumed since the project is located in a CBD area. In this vehicle mix, autos from 1975–1978 were considered to be equipped with catalytic converters, while the others were noncatalytic.
4. An average temperature of 65°F was assumed, since air pollution episodes occur most frequently during fall seasons.
5. For worst case conditions such as rush-hours or peak holiday shopping periods (1–8 hr), it was assumed that the entire vehicle population was in either a hot or cold start operating mode. For longer periods such as daily averages, the hot/cold start operational characteristics typical of a metropolitan area were utilized (5). The percent of vehicles in a particular class undergoing hot or cold starts are given in Table 13.2.

In the following sections, the data derived above is used to calculate composite emission factors for the pollutants of interest, CO, PM, SO_4, and Pb.

Table 13.1 Light-Duty, Vehicle Age, and Mileage Mix

Age	Fraction of Travel	Year
0	0.102	1978
1	0.159	1977
2	0.172	1976
3	0.130	1975
4	0.097	1974
5	0.083	1973
6	0.073	1972
7	0.058	1971
8	0.042	1970
9	0.031	1969
10	0.020	1968
11	0.011	1967
12 and over	0.015	pre-1967

Table 13.2 Percentage of Vehicles in a Particular Class Undergoing Hot or Cold Starts

Time Periods	Catalytic Vehicles	Noncatalytic Vehicles
Peak hours		
Hot starts	20%	0%
Cold starts	50%	30%
Daily average		
Hot starts	10%	0%
Cold starts	25%	14%

Carbon Monoxide

An emission factor for CO is given by the solution of

$$e_{\mathrm{CO}} = \sum_{i=n-12}^{n} c_{\mathrm{ipn}}\, m_{\mathrm{in}}\, v_{\mathrm{ips}}\, z_{\mathrm{ipt}}\, r_{\mathrm{iptw}} \tag{13.1}$$

where

e_{CO} = composite emission factor for carbon monoxide in g/vehicle-mile

n = design year for emisson calculation

c_{ipn} = mean emission factor from Table D.1-11 in AP-42 (3)

m_{in} = fraction of annual vehicle travel (Table 13.1)

v_{ips} = speed correction factor from Table D.1-23 (3)

z_{ipt} = temperature correction factor from Table D.1-26 (3) (1.124 for noncatalyst and 1.75 for catalyst)

r_{iptw} = hot/cold vehicle operation factor for noncatalytic vehicles from Table D.1-26 (3): $= [w + (100 - w)f(t)]/[20 + 80f(t)]$, where w = percent cold operation

r_{iptwx} = hot/cold vehicle operation factor for catalyst equipped vehicles $= [w + xf(t) + (100 - w - x)\,g(t)]/[20 + 27f(t) + 53g(t)]$ where w = percent cold operation and x = percent hot start operation.

$f(t)$ and $g(t)$ are temperature factors (t in degrees F) of the form e^a, where $a = 0.035t - 5.24$ for $g(t)$, $a = 0.036t - 4.14$ for $f(t)$ and catalyst equipped vehicles, and $a = 0.0045t + 0.02$ for $f(t)$ and noncatalytic vehicles.

The results of the calculation for peak periods are presented in Table 13.3. The peak period emission factor is 65.26 g/vehicle-mile, while the daily average value is 47.3 g/vehicle-mile.

Particulates and Sulfates

Data for particulate and sulfate emission variation with vehicle model year and speed is sparse. AP-42 (2,3) presents average emission factors

Table 13.3 1978 CO Composite Emission Factor Calculation

Model Year	c	m	v	z	r	e
1978	2.8	0.102	1.28	1.75	2.017	1.29
1977	9.9	0.159	"	"	"	7.11
1976	10.8	0.172	"	"	"	8.39
1975	11.7	0.130	"	"	"	6.87
1974	45.0	0.097	"	1.124	1.153	7.24
1973	47.0	0.083	"	"	"	6.47
1972	49.0	0.073	"	"	"	5.93
1971	66.0	0.058	"	"	"	6.35
1970	68.5	0.042	"	"	"	4.81
1969	80.4	0.031	"	"	"	4.13
1968	82.6	0.020	1.23	"	"	2.63
pre-1968	99.0	0.026	1.21	"	"	4.04
					e_{CO} (peak period) =	65.26 g/vehicle-mile

for all catalyst-equipped and noncatalyst vehicles. A general equation for average emission factor is:

$$e = f_{ncv}e_{ncv} + f_{cv}e_{cv} \tag{13.2}$$

where

e = composite emission factor, in this case e_{PM} for particulates and e_{SO_4} for sulfates in g/vehicle-mile
f_{ncv} = fraction of noncatalyst vehicles (0.44 in 1978)
f_{cv} = fraction of catalyst-equipped vehicles = $1 - f_{ncv}$
e_{ncv} = emission factor for noncatalyst vehicles from Table 1-21 (3)
e_{cv} = emission factor for catalyst-equipped vehicles from Table 1-21 (3).

For particulates the results are e_{PM} = 0.38 g/vehicle-mile, while for sulfates e_{SO_4} = 0.034 g/vehicle-mile.

Lead

Emission of lead from noncatalyst vehicles may be conservatively estimated by assuming that:

1. gasoline contains 2 g lead/gal
2. 70% of lead appears as tailpipe emissions
3. average vehicles get 14 miles/gal.

These considerations yield a noncatalyst emission rate of 0.1 g/vehicle-mile. The lead content permitted in fuel for catalyst-equipped cars is 0.05 g/gal. Using the other assumptions noted above, the emission rate for catalyst-equipped vehicles equals 0.0025 g/vehicle-mile.

The overall emission rate is:

$$e_{Pb} = f_{ncv}e_{ncv} + f_{cv}e_{cv} \tag{13.3}$$

where:

e_{Pb} = composite emission factor for lead, g/vehicle-mile
f_{ncv} = fraction of noncatalyst vehicles (0.44 in 1978)
f_{cv} = fraction of catalyst-equipped vehicles = $1 - f_{ncv}$
e_{ncv} = emission rate for noncatalyst vehicles = 0.1 g/vehicle-mile
e_{cv} = emission rate for catalyst-equipped vehicles = 0.0025 g/vehicle-mile.

The overall emission rate for lead e_{Pb} equals 0.045 g/vehicle-mile.

Idle Emissions

Another important consideration is the emissions produced by vehicles using the proposed parking garage. Due to the extremely low-speed nature of auto operation in a parking structure, idle emissions were used to estimate such a condition. In a garage of the size proposed (2000–2500 spaces) a peak period idling time of 5 min was assumed. This applied to both entry and exit movements during congested conditions. It was also assumed that an idling vehicle travels at the rate of 0.5 mph while entering and exiting or searching for a space. A rate of 0.5 mph over 5 min is equivalent to each vehicle traveling 0.04 mile within the garage.

To predict idle CO emissions, the EPA provides a 1974 baseline emission rate and correction factors (6). Thus

$$e_{CO} = \frac{\text{1974 baseline}}{\text{1974 factor}} \times \text{1978 factor} \tag{13.4}$$

$$= \frac{\text{16.2 g/vehicle-min}}{\text{67.5 g/vehicle-mile}} \times \text{42.7 g/vehicle-mile}$$

$$= \text{10.25 g CO/vehicle-min}$$

Based on 5 min, e_{CO} = 51.25 g CO/vehicle.

For SO_4, Pb, and PM, idle emission factors may be calculated on a distance-traveled basis:

$$\text{0.034 g } SO_4\text{/vehicle-mile} \times \text{0.04 mile} = \text{0.001 g } SO_4\text{/vehicle}$$
$$\text{0.38 g PM/vehicle-mile} \times \text{0.04 mile} = \text{0.015 g PM/vehicle}$$
$$\text{0.10 g PB/vehicle-mile} \times \text{0.04 mile} = \text{0.004 g Pb/vehicle.}$$

The emission factors derived for use in this study are summarized in Table 13.4.

Traffic Patterns

To complete the calculation of air pollutant emissions, existing and projected traffic volumes must be considered. The network volume assign-

Table 13.4 Emission Factor Summary

Pollutant	At 15 mph (g/vehicle-mile)	At 5-min Idle (g/vehicle)
CO	65.26	51.25
SO_4	0.034	0.001
PM	0.38	0.015
Pb	0.045	0.004

ments presented in Figures 13.1 and 13.2 are typical of the traffic information generated during project planning. These data are for weekday peak-hour (p.m.) and Saturday peak-hour traffic levels under both existing and proposed conditions. The data for proposed conditions, or "design level" data, were based on expected incremental traffic volume changes due to shopping activities on the fifth busiest weekday and tenth busiest Saturday of the year. It was also assumed that 57% of the shopping trips are made by auto.

Traffic network assignments must be transformed to vehicular miles traveled (VMT) for emission calculations. This is accomplished by totaling average traffic volumes over each roadway segment between intersections. The existing and design level results of VMT calculation are given in Table 13.5.

While the data given in Figures 13.1 and 13.2 are normally adequate for transportation facility planning, it is desirable to consider a wider variety of conditions in an air quality analysis. The greatest emission intensities and, consequently, the greatest health hazards are likely to occur as episodes of short duration. The relationship of air pollution episodes to health hazards is recognized in the federally promulgated air quality

Table 13.5 Existing and Projected Vehicular Miles Travelled

	Weekday (p.m.) Peak Hour	Saturday Peak Hour
Existing traffic	860 VMT	820 VMT
Projected traffic	980 VMT	1005 VMT

standards which specify measurement periods of 1, 8, and 24 hr for various pollutants at differing intensity levels.

Factors have been derived from basic traffic engineering parameters to transform the design levels into "worst case" forms compatible with episodal analysis. In general, peak-hour values may be transformed to 8-hr and 24-hr data with the following relations:

24-hr traffic	= average daily traffic (ADT)
Average peak hour	= 7.25% ADT
Worst peak hour	= 11% ADT
Average 8-hr traffic	= 48% ADT
Worst 8-hr traffic	= 60% ADT

The episodal concept was also applied to the predicted modal split of 57% of the shoppers as drivers by postulating a worst case condition of 100% drivers. Similarly, the design trip levels for the fifth highest weekday and tenth highest Saturday were projected to highest weekday and highest Saturday by using the sales effectiveness ratio. Figure 13.3 shows the case study plot of sales effectiveness ratios for the *i*th highest shopping periods. These ratios predict the number of shopping trips generated in a given period compared to a "typical" or thirtieth highest level. The adjustment from the case study design levels to the highest or "zeroth" level are given by

$$\frac{\text{highest weekday}}{\text{fifth highest weekday}} = \frac{2.15}{2.00} = 1.08$$

$$\frac{\text{highest Saturday}}{\text{tenth highest Saturday}} = \frac{2.15}{1.70} = 1.26$$

A set of basic traffic conditions for analysis were defined on the basis of the preceding relationships. Each of the conditions was evaluated at 1-hr, 8-hr, and 24-hr episodal levels for both weekdays and Saturdays. The conditions are the following:

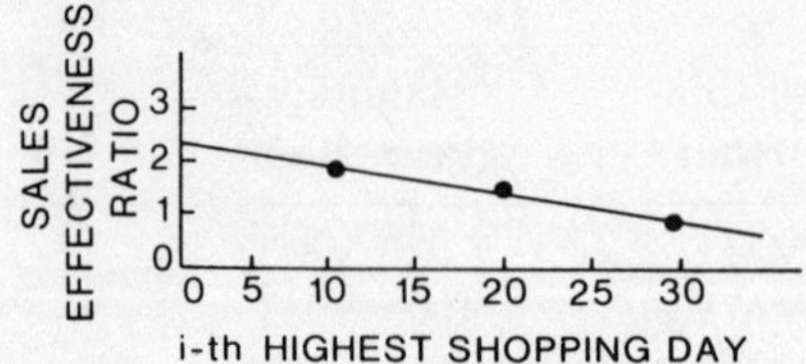

Figure 13.3. Sales effectiveness ratio for highest shopping days.

a = existing observed traffic.
b = worst case existing traffic (condition $a \times 11/7.25$ for peak hour; condition $a \times 60/7.25$ for 8 hr)
c = projected traffic generation (design level).
d = worst case traffic generation (adjusted to ''zeroth'' day' condition $c \times 1.26$ or 1.08)
e = projected traffic generation—100% driving (condition $c/0.57$—assume all shoppers drive autos)
f = worst case traffic generation—100% driving (condition $d/0.57$)

The proposed 2000-vehicle parking garage is also an important potential source of air pollutant emissions. It was analyzed for conditions similar to those designated by c–f above. However, rather than rely upon traffic network assignments, garage usage was defined on the basis of the total trip-making generated by the proposed center. This is readily available data in a design study since it forms the background for derivation of network volume assignments. In this case study the total trips were given as 1080 trips on the fifth highest weekday and 1450 trips on the tenth highest Saturday. Garage traffic movements are designated by letters g–k.

Emission Estimates

The results of applying the previously calculated composite emission factors to the vehicular travel patterns are presented in Table 13.6. These data allow estimation of gross pollutant emissions during the typical periods examined by combining the appropriate conditions. Thus existing average conditions a, or worst probable conditions b, may be compared to projected conditions after implementation $a + c + g$, or worst probable conditions with a normal modal split $b + d + h$, or worst possible conditions with 100% drivers as an ultimate case $b + f + k$.

Table 13.7 presents time-averaged emissions for 1, 8, and 24-hr periods, calculated from the peak hour data in Table 13.6 and appropriate traffic volume adjustment factors from the foregoing *Traffic Patterns* section. Note that Table 13.7 shows only the emission rates associated with Saturday afternoon peak-hour traffic, since projections indicate that the highest rates are likely to occur then rather than during weekdays. By considering these values during air quality modeling, a conservative result is assured.

Table 13.6 Total Emissions for Various Traffic Conditions

Peak Hour Condition	Weekday					Saturday				
	VMT	CO (kg)	PM (g)	SO_4 (g)	Pb (g)	VMT	CO (kg)	PM (g)	SO_4 (g)	Pb (g)
Existing observed (*a*)	860	56	327	29	86	820	53	310	28	82
Worst existing (*b*)	1290	84	490	44	129	1240	81	471	42	124
Projected generation (*c*)	120	8	46	4	12	185	12	70	6	19
Worst probable generation (*d*)	130	9	49	4	13	233	15	86	8	23
Projected generation (100% drive) (*j*)	210	14	80	7	21	325	21	124	11	33
Worst possible generation (100% drive) (*f*)	227	15	86	8	23	409	27	155	14	41
	Vehicles/Hour					Vehicles/Hour				
Garage projection (*g*)	1080	55	17	2	5	1450	74	23	2	6
Worst probable garage projection (*h*)	1166	60	18	2	5	1827	94	30	3	8
Garage projection (100% drive) (*j*)	1895	97	30	3	8	2300	118	36	3	10
Worst probable projection (100% drive) (*k*)	2046	105	32	3	9	2300	118	36	3	10

Table 13.7 Average Emissions/Hour of Carbon Monoxide, Particulates, Sulfates, and Lead for 1, 8 and/or 24-Hour Time Periods

Pollutant		Traffic Condition					
		a	*b*	*c*	*f*	*g*	*k*
CO (kg/hr)	1 hr	53	81	12	27	74	118
	8 hr	44	55	10	18	61	80
	24 hr	22	22	5	7.4	22	29
Particulates (g/hr)	24 hr	178	179	40	59	9.5	12
SO_4 (g/hr)	24 hr	16	16	3.4	5.3	0.8	1.0
Pb (g/hr)	24 hr	47	47	11	15.5	2.5	3.4

AIR QUALITY MODELING

The increase in vehicular emissions as discussed in the preceding section will, of course, yield an increase in overall air pollution concentrations within a certain distance of the proposed shopping center. The extent of the increase is dependent on many factors such as the stability of the atmosphere; horizontal wind speed and direction; the natural topography of the area as well as shape and location of man-made structures; the geometry of the area from which the increase in emissions is generated; and background levels of the pollutants already in existence. Estimates of the pollutant concentrations that may be expected at a source of air pollution and at specified distances may be made by the use of dispersion models. For this case study the Gaussian dispersion equations described by Turner (7) were used.

Diffusion Equations

In general Gaussian diffusion equations are used to describe the dispersion of an inert pollutant from a point source with a constant emission rate. The method assumes that horizontal and vertical dispersion occur in a normal distribution. The general equation form (from Chapter 8) is

$$C(x, y, z, H) = \frac{Q}{2\pi\sigma_y\sigma_z u}\left\{\exp\left[-\frac{1}{2}\left(\frac{y}{\sigma_y}\right)^2\right]\right\}\left\{\exp\left[-\frac{1}{2}\left(\frac{z+H}{\sigma_z}\right)^2\right] + \exp\left[-\frac{1}{2}\left(\frac{z-H}{\sigma_z}\right)^2\right]\right\} \quad (8.2)$$

where

C = concentration of pollutant
x, y, z = receptor location coordinates
H = effective stack height
Q = source strength
σ_y, σ_z = horizontal and vertical dispersion parameters
u = mean wind speed

The equation was simplified in this case study by assuming that the source and receptor are both at ground level and that all concentrations are equivalent to those along the plume centerline. Thus wind direction is not a factor, and H, y, and z are set equal to zero. This point source equation then reduces to

$$C = \frac{Q}{\pi \sigma_y \sigma_z u} \tag{13.5}$$

The horizontal and vertical dispersion coefficients incorporate meterological stability and downwind distance from the source.

For area sources a theoretical point source is modeled at some distance d back from the leading edge of the area source (7). The distance and horizontal dispersion coefficients are adjusted so that the plume width is equal to the width of the area source. The emission intensity at the leading edge of the area source is equal to the source strength of the area. This permits uniform application of diffusivity assumptions for both point and area sources.

The rate of pollutant dispersion is dependent upon the rate and extent of mixing in the atmosphere. The least mixing and hence the greatest concentrations of pollutant occur during stable conditions (Class F).

In this study, wind roses detailing the frequency of 3-hr periods of Class F stability were obtained. These figures indicated: 24.6% of all 3-hr periods experienced Class F stability; 5.5% of these F stability periods had wind speeds less than 0.5 m/sec, 5% between 0.5 and 1.5 m/sec, and 14.1% had winds between 1.5 and 3 m/sec. While the majority of these Class F stability periods probably occur at night, a significant number of them could occur during the peak traffic periods. This justifies using Class F stability with a 1 m/sec wind as a reasonable approximation of the worst meteorological conditions that would be found for the air quality analysis.

Other assumptions necessary to carry out diffusion analysis for the study area, over and above gross emission intensities, were as follows:

1. The source area was a square 500 meters on a side. The actual area as shown in Figure 13.2 is a rectangle approximately 400 × 600 m.
2. The area source was centered around the proposed parking facility.
3. All on-street emissions were treated as an area source contribution at ground level.
4. All parking garage emissions were treated as a point source at ground level.
5. Although wind directions vary over time, to simplify the analysis, receptors were always placed downwind from the source.
6. The population living in a circle of 1.5-km radius centered at the proposed parking garage was assumed to be at greatest risk from the proposed mall. This 1.5-km circular study area is divided into three 0.5-km-wide concentric rings.
7. Projected concentrations at 0.5 km were considered to represent typical exposures for people living within 0.5 km of the source. The concentration of 0.75 km was considered representative of the 0.5–1.0-km ring and the concentration at 1.25 km represented exposures of people between 1.0 and 1.5 km from the site. Figure 13.4 shows an overlay of these rings on the study area.
8. Dispersion coefficients for the appropriate study distance are given in Table 13.8 (7).

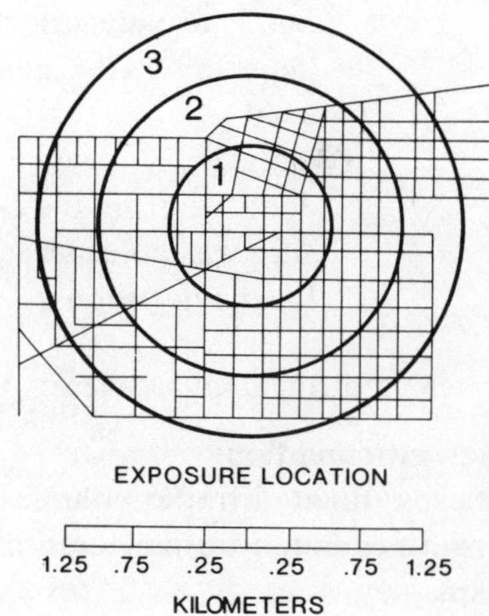

Figure 13.4. Population rings for the shopping center study area (rings centered on parking garage).

Table 13.8 Dispersion Coefficients

Distance from Center of Source Area x (km)	Virtual Distance (km)	$\sigma_y{}^a$, m		$\sigma_z{}^a$, m	
		Point	Area	Point	Area
0.5	4.30	18	128	8.4	8.5
0.75	5.55	26	135	11.5	11
1.25	5.05	42	150	16	16
1.50	5.30	50	166	18	18

[a] Class F stability assumed.

Results of Diffusion Calculations

Concentrations for the conditions and at the distances discussed above were calculated for the following time periods:

CO, 1 hr, 8 hr, 24 hr	1- and 8-hr air quality standards exist (8); 24-hr was included to enable comparison with the other 24-hr calculations
PM, 24 hr	A 24-hr air quality standard exists (8)
SO_4, 24 hr	Although no standard has been set, SO_4 is usually associated with particulates and so the same time period was used
Pb, 24 hr	Damage is based on total body burden; therefore the 24-hr average exposure was considered. A daily standard has been proposed (10).

The traffic conditions selected for analysis were:

a = existing observed conditions
b = existing highest estimated traffic volumes
c = increment from generated traffic, tenth highest shopping day, 57% auto trips
f = increment from generated traffic, highest shopping day, 100% auto trips

g = increment due to garage traffic, tenth highest shopping day, 57% auto trips

k = increment due to garage traffic, highest shopping day, 100% auto trips

Total 1 = tenth highest shopping day, 57% auto trips, $a + c + g$

Total 2 = highest shopping day, 100% auto trips, $b + f + k$

The value of Total 1 reflects pollutant concentrations on a busy traffic day and poor dispersion. The difference between Total 1 and Condition a is indicative of the incremental difference in air quality caused by the shopping center. The value of Total 2 reflects the absolute worst case (100% automobiles, poor dispersion). Results of applying the diffusion equations to the conditions above are shown in Tables 13.9 and 13.10.

Inspection of the CO data in Table 13.9 revealed unexpectedly high levels derived from the parking structure, modeled as a point source (g and k). It was decided, therefore, to model the garage as an area source, in the same manner as the general traffic circulation. This approach is believed to place reasonable upper and lower bounds upon the potential CO concentrations generated by the shopping center. The limits show that while the 1-hr standard of 40 mg/m^3 is exceeded only at the upper limit for a 0.5-km distance, the 8-hr standard of 10 mg/m^3 may be exceeded under the lower limit at 0.5 km and up to 1.25 km at the upper limit (Table 13.11). Adjustments were not made for other pollutants since the quantities emitted from the garage were relatively minor.

RECEPTORS

Certain populations are known to be more susceptible to the adverse effects of pollutants than other groups. For example, people with respiratory problems generally are more sensitive to ozone pollution than are normally healthy individuals. Young children are sensitive to all pollutants because of their high metabolic rate. Although prediction of health effects corresponding to different levels of concentration of a specific pollutant is difficult and sometimes imprecise, it is possible to identify and enumerate some of the groups potentially at risk from pollutants generated by a new installation. The types, numbers, and locations of the susceptible groups found within the study area are presented in the following section.

Table 13.9 Carbon Monoxide Concentrations for Various Distances and Traffic Conditions[a]

Ring	Distance (km)		Traffic Condition a	b	c	f	g	k	Total 1 $=a+c+g$	Total 2 $=b+f+k$	Total 1 $-a$
		1 hr	4.3	6.6	1.0	2.2	43.0	69.0	48.3	77.8	44.0
1	0.5	8 hr	3.5	4.5	0.8	1.5	35.8	47.0	40.1	53.0	36.6
		24 hr	1.8	1.8	0.4	0.6	12.9	17.0	15.1	19.4	13.3
		1 hr	3.2	4.8	0.7	1.6	21.9	34.9	25.8	41.3	22.6
2	0.75	8 hr	2.6	3.3	0.6	1.1	18.1	23.8	21.3	28.2	18.7
		24 hr	1.3	1.3	0.3	0.4	6.5	8.6	8.1	10.3	6.8
		1 hr	2.0	3.0	0.4	1.0	9.8	15.1	12.2	19.1	10.2
3	1.25	8 hr	1.6	2.0	0.4	0.7	8.0	10.6	10.0	13.3	8.4
		24 hr	0.8	0.8	0.2	0.3	2.9	3.8	3.9	4.4	3.1
		1 hr	1.8	2.7	0.4	0.9	7.2	11.6	9.4	15.2	7.6
	1.50	8 hr	1.5	1.8	0.3	0.6	6.0	7.9	7.8	10.3	6.3
		24 hr	0.8	0.8	0.2	0.2	2.2	5.7	3.2	6.7	2.4

[a] Concentrations in mg/m^3.

Table 13.10 Twenty-Four Hour Concentrations of Lead, Sulfate and Particulate Matter for Various Distances and Traffic Conditions[a]

Ring	Distance (km)		Traffic Conditions a	b	c	f	g	k	Total 1 $=a+c+g$	Total 2 $=b+f+k$	Total 1 $-a$
		Pb	1.7	1.7	0.4	0.6	0.7	0.9	2.8	3.2	1.1
1	0.5	SO_4	1.3	1.3	0.3	0.4	0.5	0.6	2.1	2.3	0.8
		PM	14.5	14.5	3.3	4.8	5.5	7.1	23.3	26.4	8.8
		Pb	1.3	1.3	0.3	0.4	0.3	0.4	1.9	2.1	0.6
2	0.75	SO_4	1.0	1.0	0.2	0.3	0.2	0.3	1.4	1.6	0.4
		PM	10.6	10.7	2.4	3.5	2.8	3.6	15.8	17.8	5.2
		Pb	0.8	0.8	0.2	0.3	0.2	0.2	1.2	1.3	0.4
3	1.24	SO_4	0.6	0.6	0.1	0.2	0.1	0.1	0.8	0.9	0.2
		PM	6.6	6.6	1.5	2.2	1.2	1.6	9.3	10.4	2.7
		Pb	0.7	0.7	0.2	0.2	0.1	0.2	1.0	1.1	0.3
	1.50	SO_4	0.5	0.5	0.1	0.2	0.2	0.1	0.8	0.8	0.3
		PM	6.0	6.0	1.4	2.0	0.9	1.2	8.3	9.2	2.3

[a] Concentrations in $\mu g/m^3$.

Table 13.11 Carbon Monoxide Concentrations for Parking Garage Modeled as an Area Source[a]

Distance (km)	Time (hr)	Traffic Conditions *a*	*c*	g^{*b}	*g*	Lower Limit[c]	Upper Limit[d]
0.5	1	4.3	1.0	6.0	43.0	11.3	48.3
	8	3.5	0.8	5.0	35.8	9.3	40.1
0.75	1	3.2	0.7	4.4	21.9	8.3	25.8
	8	2.6	0.7	3.6	18.1	6.9	21.4
1.25	1	2.0	0.4	2.7	9.8	5.1	12.2
	8	1.6	0.4	2.2	8.0	4.2	10.0
1.5	1	1.8	0.4	2.5	7.2	4.7	9.4
	8	1.5	0.3	2.0	6.0	3.8	7.8

[a] Concentrations in mg/m^3.
[b] g* models garage as 0.5-km square area source.
[c] $a + c + g^*$ = lower limit.
[d] Models garage as a point source, $a + c + g$ = Total 1 = upper limit.

Sources of Data and Enumeration Procedures

Information on the total population, number of persons over age 62, and children less than age 5 in the study area was gathered from the 1970 census. Census blocks were assigned to the study rings according to geographic area. Population per ring was thus obtained by summing over all blocks assigned to that ring.

The population of persons less than 5 years of age was not available from block statistics, but was obtained indirectly by the formula

$$S_i = \sum_{j=1}^{n} E_{ij} TP_{ij} CT_{ik} \tag{13.6}$$

where

S_i = total persons less than 5 years of age located within ring i
E_{ij} = proportion of total population in block j located in ring i
TP_{ij} = total population for block j
CT_{ik} = proportion of those under 18 years who are less than 5 years residing in census tract k within which block j is located

Equation 13.6 assumes that the proportion of all persons under 18 years of age who are less than 5 years old is the same for both the census block and census tract within which that census block is located. This may not be the case as the actual proportion for each block is likely to be somewhat greater or less than the overall proportion for the census tract, depending on the geographic distribution of 5 year olds. However, since data for many blocks must be summed to find a total for a given ring, the formula probably gives a good approximation of the number of persons less than 5 years who were located within each of the rings in 1970.

Information on enrollments in elementary schools was obtained from the local school district. The State Department of Public Health provided information on long-term care facilities and hospitals in the area. Other local groups were able to provide enrollment data for nurseries, day-care centers and senior citizen centers.

Note that the information based on census data is for 1970. Obviously, none of those persons under 5 years of age in 1970 are under 5 years in 1978. The number of elderly (over 62) may have decreased or increased depending on the healthiness of those over 62 and the number of persons 57–62 years of age in 1970. Total population probably did not change very much in the area from 1970 to 1978 because very little open land was available for development in 1970. Applying general population trends, the number of persons over 62 years might be expected to have slightly decreased from 1970 to 1978. In addition to age-based receptor groups, there are those persons who are hypersusceptible to pollutants on the basis of preexisting pathological conditions. This group includes, for example, asthmatics, bronchitics, and persons with emphysema or heart disease. The number of these hypersusceptibles was determined from a statistical high-risk population estimation technique (9). Table 13.12 summarizes the populations of hypersusceptibles considered to be at risk from the pollutants studied.

EFFECTS ON POPULATIONS AT RISK

Lead

Lead has long been recognized as a health hazard, traditionally associated with central nervous system effects. As a metabolic poison lead causes affected cells to use oxygen inefficiently. Lead is regarded as a poison that can accumulate in the body, and the contribution of inhaled lead to the

Table 13.12 Some Population Groups at High Risk to Pollutant Exposures by Distance from the Pollutant Source Area

	Ring		
Susceptible Group	1	2	3
Total population	4,959	12,530	13,227
Children under 5 years old	155	724	912
Day-care centers/nurseries	72	146	190
Elementary schools	0	672	1,006
Hospital beds	44	0	56
Long-term care beds	110	60	5
Population over 62 years	995	2,757	1,658
Asthmatics (total for the whole area)		920	
Persons with emphysema (total for the whole area)		600	
Bronchitics (total for the whole area)		950	
Persons with heart disease (total for the whole area)		716	

body burden is not insubstantial even at low exposure (e.g., 1.5 $\mu g/m^3$) (10). Children are particularly susceptible to lead effects. There is evidence that low-level lead exposures in children are capable of producing behavioral disorders, learning disability, and changes in heme synthesis. A number of studies have suggested that lead emitted from automobiles is a health hazard to children. One study has found a relationship between elevated blood lead levels (a measure of lead body burden) and traffic volume in children 1–5 years old residing near heavy traffic density (11). Other subclinical effects are summarized in Chapter 6.

The area near the proposed shopping center contains a significant number of population groups considered at risk from lead. Almost 1800 children under 5 years reside in the 1.5-km radius area around the shopping center. Lead levels on the tenth worst shopping day of the year, with 57% of the shoppers driving, may average 1–3 μg Pb/m^3 depending on the distance from the center (Tables 13.10 and 13.12).

The Environmental Health Resource Center in Illinois has recommended a standard of 1.5 μg of lead/m^3 for a 24-hr average (10). If emissions estimated in Table 13.10 were to prevail on weekdays, children spending their days attending elementary schools, day-care centers, and nurseries may be exposed to lead levels well above 1.5 $\mu g/m^3$. Almost 700 children attend K–8 schools only 0.75 km from the center, where they may be exposed to 24-hr average levels of over 2 $\mu g/m^3$. Of additional concern are 70 toddlers who attend a day-care center at a distance of 0.5 km from the center where Pb levels may reach 3 $\mu g/m^3$.

Sulfates and Particulates

As has been discussed in Chapter 4, population groups susceptible to PM and sulfates include the elderly, young children, and those with preexisting diseases of the heart and preexisting lung diseases such as asthma, chronic bronchitis, and emphysema.

The current federal standard for particulates is 260 $\mu g/m^3$ for a 24-hr average and 75 $\mu g/m^3$ for an annual average (8). Table 13.10 shows that under worst case conditions only 23.3 $\mu g/m^3$ or 10% of the 24-hr standard could be generated by the shopping center. There are no current federal, state, or local standards for SO_4.

The sulfate and particulate concentrations generated by the development are below levels that have been correlated with adverse health affects (12–14). However, the impact of other sources of these pollutants have not been included in the air quality analysis. It is possible, therefore, that the development in combination with other sources could have an adverse impact to susceptible people living in the area.

Based on the 1970 census and a high-risk population estimation technique (9), there are approximately 920 asthmatics, 950 bronchitics, and 600 people with emphysema living within 1.5 km of the proposed shopping center who might be affected by the increased SO_4 and particulates shown on Table 13.10. In addition, Table 13.12 shows 1791 children $\leq$ 5 years of age, 408 nursery school children, and 1678 elementary school children who might be harmed by incremental increases in sulfates and particulates.

Carbon Monoxide

As was discussed in Chapter 6, exposure to carbon monoxide results in reduction of the oxygen supply to various organs. Groups most suscepti-

Table 13.13 Predicted Carboxyhemoglobin Levels in Nonsmokers for Various Distances and Traffic Conditions[a]

Distance from Center of Study Area (km)	Traffic Condition		
	(a)	Total 1	Total 2
0.5	≤ 1.0	4.6	6.0
0.75	< 1.0	2.2	3.5
1.25	< 1.0	1.7	1.9
1.50	< 1.0	1.2	1.5

[a] Percent COHb for 8-hr exposure; for smokers, levels may be higher by 4% COHb.

ble to the toxic effects of CO are infants and persons with cardiovascular disease, anemia, lung disease, and/or increased metabolic rate (15).

The U.S. EPA has established CO standards of 40 mg/m³ for 1 hr and 10 mg/m³ averaged over 8 hr, not to be exceeded more than once per year (8). These standards are based primarily upon impairment of time-interval discrimination, psychomotor functions, and visual discriminization, and upon physiologic stress on heart patients. As shown in Table 13.9, the 1-hr standard may be exceeded at up to 0.75 km from the shopping center under the worst possible conditions. Similarly, the 8-hr standard may be exceeded at up to 1.5 km.

The effect of CO upon humans is reflected by the level of carboxyhemoglobin (COHb) present in the blood. In Table 13.13 some example COHb levels for nonsmokers exposed to CO concentrations for the existing and proposed traffic conditions are shown. These levels have been calculated from the theoretical CFK equation discussed in Chapter 6 and Figure 6.1. The health implications of increased COHb levels were outlined in Chapter 6.

SUMMARY

The results of this study predict a decrease in overall air quality within 1.5 km of the new shopping mall. This change in air quality could have an adverse impact on a total of 30,700 residents, of which 10,000 persons are identified as hypersensitive to air pollution.

Potential violations of ambient air quality standards for CO have been identified for distances up to 1.25 km from the center. Evidence for concern over Pb, sulfate and particulate levels has also been raised. Given the fact that numerous simplifying assumptions and data approximations have been utilized, the results still highlight the need for detailed study of any project of this type and magnitude. Air quality considerations clearly must form an essential part of project planning. Emphasis should be placed upon minimizing dependence upon the automobile for trip making, reduction of vehicular idling times, and attention to the proximity of hypersusceptible population groups during site selection and project design.

REFERENCES

1. Hallenbeck, W., Hankett, R., Hesse, C., Holden, J., Kunze, R., Neal, A., Scheff, P., and Wadden, R. *Evaluation of Potential Air Quality Impact of the Westcor Development on Evanston, Illinois*. University of Illinois School of Public Health Report, November 1976.
2. U.S. Environmental Protection Agency. *Compilation of Air Pollutant Emission Factors*, 2nd ed., AP-42, 1973.
3. U.S. Environmental Protection Agency. *Compilation of Air Pollutant Emission Factors*, 2nd Ed., Supplement No. 5, 1975.
4. U.S. Environmental Protection Agency, Office of Transportation and Land Use Policy. *Mobile Source Emission Factors: Interim Document*, June 1977.
5. Illinois Department of Transportation. *Air Quality Manual, Appendix B*, revised April 1976.
6. U.S. Environmental Protection Agency. *Interim Guidelines for the Review of the Impact of Indirect Sources on Ambient Air Quality*. July 1974, p. E-7.
7. Turner, B. D. *Workbook of Atmospheric Dispersion Estimates*. U.S. Department of Health, Education, and Welfare, 1970, pp. 39–40, 52.
8. U.S. Environmental Protection Agency. National primary and secondary air quality standards. *Fed. Regist.* **36:**8186, 1971.
9. Farley, D. O. *Estimation of Local Area Populations with Chronic Obstructive Lung Diseases*. MS Thesis, University of Illinois. 1976.
10. Environmental Health Resource Center. *Health Effects and Recommendations for Atmospheric Lead, Cadmium, Mercury, and Asbestos*. Illinois Institute for Environmental Quality Document No. 73-2, March 1973.
11. Caprio, R. J., Margulis, H. T., and Joselow, M. M. Lead absorption in children and its relationship to urban traffic densities. *Arch. Environ. Health*, **28:**195–197, 1974.

12. Carnow, B. W., Lepper, M. H., Shekelle, R. B., and Stamler, J. Chicago air pollution study: SO_2 levels and acute illness in patients with chronic bronchopulmonary disease. *Arch. Environ. Health*, **18**:768–776, 1969.
13. Shy, C. M., Hasselblad, V., Burton, R. M., Nelson, C. J., and Cohen, A. A. Air pollution effects on ventilatory function of U.S. school children. Results of studies in Cincinnati, Chattanooga, and New York. *Arch. Environ. Health*, **27**:124–128, 1973.
14. U.S. Environmental Protection Agency. *Health Consequences of Sulfur Oxides: A Report from CHESS, 1970–1971*. EPA-650/1-74-004, U.S. Government Printing Office, Washington, DC, May 1974.
15. Stewart, R. D. The effect of carbon monoxide on humans. *J. Occup. Med.*, **18**:304–309, 1976.

14

COAL HYDROGENATION EVALUATION

Janet A. Holden and Richard A. Wadden

The most abundant energy resource in the United States is coal. Identified deposits that are recoverable with present technology are calculated to be 12–19 times greater than U.S. petroleum reserves (1). In 1974 the 600 million tons of coal produced accounted for only 18% of total U.S. energy consumption. However, the use of coal for energy is projected to increase substantially over the next few decades, and production could reach over 1 billion tons by 1985 (2). Because of the demand for low-sulfur, environmentally acceptable fuels, conversion of coal to synthetic fuels through coal hydrogenation is being investigated. The technology for the hydrogenation process by coal liquefaction or gasification has been demonstrated on a commercial scale in Germany, England, and South Africa. Environmental measurements from these plants, however, were either not made or are not available.

COAL HYDROGENATION

At present, no commercial scale liquefaction or gasification plants exist in the United States. There are some plants in the planning stages and a number of pilot plants either are operating or have been demonstrated. Evaluation of the potential environmental effects of coal processing depends on data from these pilot plants and from bench scale reactors.

Commercially feasible gasification plant sizes will typically convert in excess of 20,000 tons/day of coal into products and wastes (3). Because of the large amounts of material being processed, the potential exists for environmental discharge of considerable quantities of hazardous materials. These include hydrogen cyanide, phenols, cresols, carbonyl and hydrogen sulfides, ammonia, mercaptans, thiocyanides, aniline, arsenic, trace metals, and various polycyclic hydrocarbons (3–8).

Sources of possible pollution from hydrogenation plants can generally be classified into three categories: the nature of the raw material, the design of the processing scheme, and the way in which the process is actually operated (3). Coal has a very complex, heterocyclic structure, which must be broken down to produce desirable products (see Figure 7.1). A given coal conversion process will destroy many of these bonds. Thiophene, methylpyridine, hydroxynapthalene, and benzo(a)pyrene are only a few of the compounds that could reasonably be expected to be produced. However, the cleavage of these cyclic linkages and the chemical form of the resultant compounds are difficult to analyze and predict. As is indicated in Tables 14.1 and 14.2, coal also contains significant quantities of hazardous metals and considerable amounts of sulfur and nitrogen (3,9). For example, arsenic, beryllium, mercury, lead, and vanadium have all been identified as materials with properties toxic to man (10). Functional groups in coal include the methoxy, hydroxyl, carbonyl, and carboxyl groups. These can lead to the formation of contaminants and hazards such as phenols, metal carbonyls, aromatic nitrogen, and sulfur compounds (3).

Many different coal hydrogenation processes have been attempted or projected. Each must be analyzed specifically for the types of wastes produced and how they are distributed to water, air, and soil. However, some general observations can be made about the nature of the conversion process. Most hydrogenation processes require elevated temperatures and pressures in order to break down the coal. Table 14.3 indicates the atomic hydrogen to carbon ratios of various raw materials and finished

Table 14.1 Some Trace Elements in Coal and Coal Gasifier Gas (3)

	Concentration (lb of trace element/1000 tons of coal)	
Element	Coal	Coal Gasifier Gas
As	28.0	27.7
B	204.0	97.3
Be	3.2	0.1
Cd	5.0	
Co	19.1	
Cr	27.5	
Cu	30.3	
F	122.0	121.0
Hg	0.4	0.4
Mn	98.8	6.8
Mo	15.1	13.7
Ni	42.1	
Pb	69.6	25.2
Sb	2.5	1.9
Se	4.2	
Sn	9.6	
V	65.4	
Zr	145.0	

products (3). The energy to generate the necessary heat is ordinarily derived from oxidizing a portion of the incoming coal. Hydrogen is supplied either through direct or indirect utilization of the hydrogen atoms in water or through use of a hydrogen donor solvent.

In a typical coal gasification plant, the coal is first ground, dried, and preheated and then fed to a gasification unit. In the gasification step the coal is reacted with steam to yield carbon monoxide and hydrogen. The hydrogen then reacts further with the coal to yield gas with a low heating value (approximately 200 Btu/ft^3) and char. In order to obtain pipeline gas (approximately 950 Btu/ft^3) further conversion is required. In the shift reaction carbon monoxide is reacted with more steam over a catalyst to yield hydrogen. In the methanation step carbon monoxide reacts with the hydrogen to yield a hydrogen-rich high-Btu product gas. The major reactions are:

$C(coal) + H_2O \rightarrow CO + H_2$ gasification reaction

$C(coal) + H_2 \rightarrow CH_4$ + char (low Btu value)

$CO + H_2O(Steam) \xrightarrow[cat.]{} CO_2 + H_2$ shift reaction

$CO + 3H_2 \xrightarrow[cat.]{} CH_4 + H_2O$ (~ 950 Btu/ft^3) methanation reaction

The product gas is cleaned of H_2S and NH_3, and the hydrogen is removed and recycled to the reaction step. The liquid products are distilled to yield light and heavy fuel oil products. Sulfur and ammonia are also formed in marketable quantities.

Temperatures of 700–1000°F and pressures up to 1500 psig are needed for hydrogenation. The specific operating conditions will determine what gaseous and solid byproducts are formed, as well as the product ratios of

Table 14.2 Chemical Analysis of Typical Illinois No. 6 Coal (3)

	Concentration (tons/1000 tons dry coal)
Carbon	707
Hydrogen	54
Nitrogen	10
Sulfur	50
Oxygen	80
Ash	99

Table 14.3 Hydrogen/Carbon Atomic Ratios in Typical Fuels (3)

Fuel	Atomic ratio H/C
Coal (Illinois No. 6)	0.86
Heating oil	
Residual (No. 6)	1.55
Distillate (No. 2)	1.79
Naphtha	2.20
LPG	2.65
Natural gas	3.40
Pure methane	4.00

gas to liquid. This type of coal processing yields enormous quantities of waste products and heat. The products are formed directly as gases, solids, or liquids and are cleaned out of the waste streams by means of water treatment or such waste removal processes as scrubbers, cyclones, and bag houses. Each treatment process, of course, yields final waste products.

Waste char and ash, which require disposal, amount to 20–30% of the raw coal input (3). Some phenolic material is likely to be disposed of with the waste ash and char and has the potential to be leached out into water systems (6). A variety of catalysts, including compounds containing iron, zinc, aluminum, copper, and cobalt, are used in coal hydrogenation (11). Perhaps of greatest concern are the types utilized for methanation in the gasification process. Nickel, cobalt, iron, rubidium, osmium, and platinum have all been suggested as possible catalysts. The presence of nickel carbonyl [$Ni(CO)_4$] (a suspected carcinogen (12)) has been reported in methanizer product gas (13). Since temperatures less than 525°F encourage the formation of $Ni(CO)_4$ and reduced conversion of carbon monoxide to methane, careful temperature control is necessary for process as well as health reasons. In certain industrial settings platinum and palladium have been implicated in the occurrence of an asthmalike disease, although their existence in the gas phase in significant concentrations is problematical (14,15).

Heavy oil and tars produced by hydrogenation may comprise a quantity of 30,000–200,000 lb/1000 tons coal or 300–2000 tons/day in a commercial size plant (3). At present, these materials are not completely characterized. A partial analysis of some of the constituents contained in the tar from a gasification pilot plant is shown in Table 14.4. It has been sug-

Table 14.4 Some Tar Constituents in the Synthane Coal-to-Gas Process (3,5)

	Concentration (vol %)
Naphthalene	11.6
Fluorenes	9.6
Three-ring aromatics	13.8
Phenols	4.0
N-Heterocyclics	10.8

gested that the heavy oils can be used (and consequently controlled) by recycling them to the main hydrogenation reactor for further reduction and/or by using them to slurry the incoming coal (3). However, there is evidence that some materials of higher molecular weight may not be completely degraded (16). In addition, product liquids may have higher aromatic contents than naturally occurring hydrocarbons with the same boiling point characteristics (17). Since many cyclic hydrocarbons have been identified as hazardous to man, the potential of these liquids for causing adverse effects on the central nervous system, liver, kidneys, and skin, as well as their possible carcinogenicity, should be analyzed.

Only one study of the actual health hazards of coal hydrogenation is presently available (6,8,16,18). A group of 359 workers was examined for skin cancer over a period of 5 years at a pilot liquefaction plant designed to process 300 tons/day of incoming coal. Of this group, 10 men developed skin cancer. Exposure varied from several months to 23 years, but all significant lesions were found in workers with less than 10 years of exposure. The reported incidence was 16–37 times the incidence of skin cancer expected in the chemical industry (18). Analyses of the liquid materials produced in the plant identified a number of carcinogenic materials. An increase in carcinogenicity with increasing liquid boiling point, usually with respect to liquids with boiling points greater than 260°C (500°F), was observed in laboratory animals (16). This relationship was particularly evident for the oil produced in the plant that was recycled to slurry the incoming coal. In addition, air measurements in working areas revealed benzo(a)pyrene concentrations often in excess of 50 $\mu g/1000\ m^3$ with a peak value of 18,000 $\mu g/1000\ m^3$ (6). Benzo(a)pyrene has been identified as being strongly carcinogenic (19). These concentrations are in contrast to typical urban levels of 3–6 $\mu g/1000\ m^3$ (19).

Health statistics on occupational groups in other coal conversion operations, such as coke ovens and coal-tar processing, have shown significantly higher lung cancer rates relative to groups without such occupational exposures (19–22). In particular, coke oven workers appear to have 2.5 times the incidence of lung cancer as other steel workers (21). The environment on top of a coke oven is, of course, different from that likely to occur in hydrogenation plants that process material continuously. There is no assurance that the same incidence of cancer or any other disease will occur. However, close control of environmental discharges is strongly suggested in light of these occupational observations and the hydrogenation plant data cited above.

EXAMPLE OF EVALUATION METHODS

The following example shows how the evaluatory framework discussed in previous chapters is applied to evaluate an Environmental Analysis Report (EAR) (23) for a proposed demonstration coal hydrogenation plant. This EAR was prepared as a preliminary document by which the decision is made whether or not to prepare a full Environmental Impact Statement. The evaluation technique presented here provided a method to point out those areas that were lacking and what information was still needed for a comprehensive worthwhile Impact Statement.

To accurately determine the environmental impact of the proposed coal hydrogenation plant, a minimum of three steps had to be accomplished in the EAR:

1. Identification and quantification of amounts of hazardous materials that might be discharged from the plant.
2. Estimation of possible dispersion of these materials in air and water.
3. Identification and enumeration of populations who might be exposed to discharges and determination of their exposures.

In order to accomplish these three steps the following information is needed from the EAR:

1. The amounts and composition of the plant's input and output streams.
2. Process flow diagrams with temperatures, pressures, flow rates, and compositions for each stream. (The analysis of such flow diagrams identifies the locations where the greatest degree of control is required.)
3. The amounts of hazardous materials produced and the types and efficiency levels of control equipment.
4. Historical meteorological and hydrological data for the surrounding area.
5. Historical air, water, and soil pollutant values for the surrounding areas, as well as types and location of other major pollutant sources.
6. Population densities and locations, as well as enumeration of special subgroups, such as children and the elderly.

The EAR was examined to determine what information was provided, and what additional information is still needed in each category, in order to adequately determine the environmental impact of the proposed plant.

Plant Input and Output Streams

Analyses of the types of raw coal projected for use in the hydrogenation plant were not included in the EAR. As a result no determinations could be made of possible trace element discharge to air, water, or soil. In addition, data on sulfur levels of incoming coal were conflicting in different sections of the EAR. Consequently the discharge of sulfur to the environment could not be accurately determined.

The other major feedstock is water. The EAR did include extensive information about the quality and quantity of the water to be used. This information was obtained from state agencies as well as by independent testing. The testing samples were taken from only three locations, one time each in September, November, and December. This sampling protocol did not give an accurate representation of water quality changes throughout the year. For example, it ignored the problems of summer low flows and increased agricultural runoff carrying fertilizers and pesticides during spring rains.

Other feedstocks to be used were (in the order listed in the EAR) air, nitrogen, lime, alum, H_2SO_4, caustic, chlorine. The amounts of each of these substances and their uses were unclear. Their potential chemical reactivities as well as intermediate and ultimate forms when released into the environment were not discussed.

The composition of the final products was not well defined. Specifically, the amounts of hydrogen in the product gases and the energy values for all products were not given. There was no mention of ammonia in any of the lists of final products and yet, in a general description of the process, the production of saleable ammonia was reported. Whether or not ammonia will be produced, during which steps, and wastes or byproducts formed as a result of production, should be clarified.

Process Description

The EAR contained a very general and confusing description of the processes to be used in the plant. Only vague references to "required pressures" or "high enough temperatures" were included. The composition of the streams between the different units were not specified and no flow rates or quantities were given. Figure 14.1, from the EAR, shows the

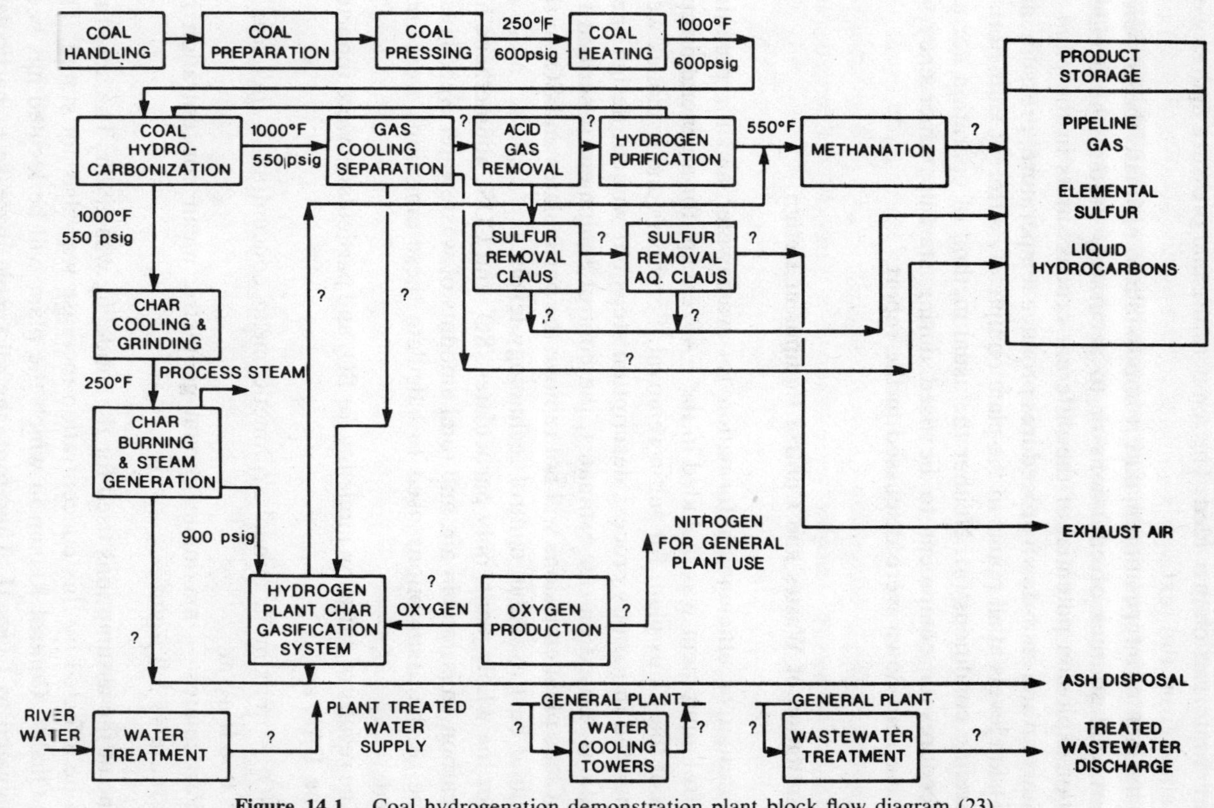

Figure 14.1. Coal hydrogenation demonstration plant block flow diagram (23).

level of information provided. The temperature and pressure figures were obtained from the text.

This lack of information makes it impossible to estimate the amounts, types, and sources of emissions or to accurately predict the accident and/or explosion potential of the different process units in the plant.

Start-up and shut-down procedures produce temperature, pressure, and emission levels at all points in the plant completely different from normal operating conditions (3). Neither the usual method of operation nor any procedures or equipment to be used during start-up, emergency, or routine shut-down were discussed in the report.

Quantitation of Wastes and Control Equipment Design

No design or efficiency information for wastewater and air pollution control equipment was included in the EAR except for a general discussion of the Claus plant for sulfur removal. Scrubbers and cyclones were mentioned in various process description steps but without design specifications. Based on our estimates, the control equipment described for the Claus plant emissions will not remove the particulates and SO_2 to the required best available control technology levels.

For the whole plant, only particulates, SO_2 and COS, nonmethane hydrocarbon emissions in air, and total amounts of wastewater were given. None of the assumptions used to calculate these emissions were indicated.

The results of diffusion modeling for SO_2 and particulates were reported in the EAR as:

1. SO_2 – maximum annual arithmetic mean concentration increase = 5.0–6.0 $\mu g/m^3$
2. Particulates – maximum annual geometric mean concentration increase = 5.0 $\mu g/m^3$

None of the assumptions used for the modeling was given. The area that will be affected by this concentration increase was also not stated. The Air Quality Control Region in which the plant will be located has been designated as Class II. Therefore, the allowable increase in particulate concentration from all sources is limited to 10 $\mu g/m^3$ and the increase for SO_2 is limited to 15 $\mu g/m^3$ (24). The preliminary modeling results, although unexplained and unsupported, indicated that emissions from the plant will use one-half of the allowable particulate increment increase and one-third of the allowable SO_2 increment increase. It appears that higher control efficiencies than those assumed in the modeling will probably be required. These increased concentrations are especially important in light of the fact that this is a demonstration plant, approximately one-fourth of the size of the proposed commercial scale plant.

The amounts and types of solid waste to be produced by the plant were not addressed in the report. Brief mention was made of the solids from the waste treatment units and an estimated 400–450 tons/day of flyash. No characterizations of these potentially hazardous materials were attempted. When we carried out detailed elemental balances, significant discrepancies between plant input and output data were encountered.

Sulfur

A crude mass balance for sulfur was considered essential in view of the potential adverse health effects of sulfur emissions. The average of the sulfur content listed in the feedstocks was used, a value of 3.3% sulfur by weight. The mass balance is given in Table 14.5. The fate of the unaccounted sulfur (1.3 tons/day) was unclear from the report. A more basic question, however, is how the SO_2 and COS emissions were estimated from the given range of sulfur input levels. Furthermore, there was no mention of the amount of anhydrous sodium sulfate produced as a byproduct of the sulfur removal process. The possibility of H_2S, SO_2, or sulfate aerosol emissions from the aqueous Claus plant was also not addressed. The amount of sulfur possibly present in the wastewater was not estimated.

Table 14.5 Sulfur Balance

Material	Tons/Day	Sulfur Fraction	Sulfur (tons/day)
Input			
Coal	3,850	0.033	127.0
Output			
Liquid sulfur product	122	1.000	122.0
SO_2 from Claus plant	7.2	0.500	3.6
COS from hydrogen plant	0.2	0.505	0.1
Total output			125.7
Unaccounted sulfur			1.3

Carbon

The proposed plant will convert the highly complex coal molecular structure into simpler hydrocarbon fuels. Its main concept involves hydrogenation of the organic fraction of coal with extensive severing of carbon-carbon and carbon-heteroatom bonds to form simple hydrocarbons. Therefore, carbon content conservation is a significant measure of the plant efficiency. That portion of the carbon not transformed to product represents a potential source of air and water contamination. A carbon balance is shown in Table 14.6. As is indicated in the table almost 1700 tons/day carbon are unaccounted for.

Other elements

Some of the trace elements that may be present in coal are presented in Table 14.2. The fate of these and any other trace materials such as those used as catalysts was not considered in the EAR.

Mass balances

Because of the amount of missing information, complete mass balances were not possible. It is clear from the sulfur and carbon balances alone that a vast quantity of material is unaccounted for in the project description. Most of this is made up of water, but a coal balance shows that some of this material is also missing. (See Table 14.7.)

Table 14.6 Carbon Balance

Material	Tons/Day	Carbon Fraction	Carbon (tons/day)
Input			
Coal	3,850	0.71	2,733.5
Output			
Heavy fuel oil	550	0.89	489.5
Light hydrocarbons	165	0.84	138.6
LPG	96	0.82	78.7
SNG	425	0.78	331.5
Air emissions			
C_2	0.3	0.80	0.2
C_3	0.6	0.82	0.5
Total output			1,039.0
Unaccounted carbon			1,694.5

Table 14.7 Coal Balance

Coal	Tons/Day
Input	
Moisture (9.0%)	346
Ash (9.3%)	359
Sulfur (3.3%)	127
Carbon (71.0%)	2,733
Other (7.3%)	285
Total in	3,850
Output	
Flyash (250–400 tons/day)	359
Sulfur	126
Moisture (8% removed)	318.3
Particulates	1.8
Carbon in products	1,037.5
Carbon for H_2 production	1,257
Carbon in air emissions	0.8
Carbon for plant energy	437.7
Solids in wastewater	6.4
Total out	3,544.5
Unaccounted coal	305.5

Attempts to carry out a water balance for the plant were not successful. The only quantities specified were 4.6 million gal/day (mgd) input, 0.61 mgd wastewater output, and 4 mgd consumed for boiler feed and process water. Since we estimated that the hydrogen needs of the plant would be satisfied by only 0.45 mgd of process water, there remains about 3.5 mgd unaccounted for. If the water evaporates from the cooling towers, it would seem that such a large quantity may create severe problems such as ground fogs and local weather alterations. The combination of large quantities of water vapor with particulates, carbon dioxide, SO_2, and sulfates is of serious concern with respect to acid rain.

Some of the possible elements to be discharged in the wastewater output were indicated in the EAR, but were not quantitated. Projected water effluent quality in terms of physical/chemical parameters was listed, but the method and assumptions used to develop the projections were not.

Energy balances

It was not possible to construct an accurate energy balance from the information in the EAR. Development of such a balance would require accurate heating values of all products, a typical mix of coals to be used and heating values of those coals, energy requirements of all processes in the proposed plant, and a complete listing of all temperatures and pressures throughout the plant.

Meteorological and Hydrological Data

In order to accurately estimate the effects of air and water contaminants emitted by any new pollutant source, the existing conditions in the area must be evaluated.

The EAR presented and analyzed meteorological data for the past 20 years for the area surrounding the proposed plant. These data included temperature, windspeed and direction, amount of precipitation, and the percentage of time that inversions, fog, and smog were present. In addition, the microclimate for the immediate plant site was analyzed using information on topography, vegetation, and hydrology. The tornado risk at the site was also calculated. If the appropriate emission data had been provided, this historical information would have been useful for dispersion calculations. Other information needed for truly accurate modeling of pollutant levels would be the percentage of time each stability class is experienced in the area.

Extensive hydrological data were also provided. This includes drainage of surface water and surface water availability, regional groundwater patterns, and the effect of strip-mining on the groundwater in the immediate vicinity of the proposed plant. Again, more information is needed to put these data to use.

Ambient Pollutant Values and other Pollutant Sources in the Area

Air

Air pollutant levels for the Air Quality Control Region in which the plant would be located were listed in the EAR. National Air Surveillance Network data and measurements taken by the local power company were utilized. However, no information was given as to sampling times or frequency. Air quality sampling at the plant site was carried out for a 1-week period. The information gathered during that time is of limited value since it is neither representative of seasonal fluctuations, nor does it provide enough of a base from which to calculate annual average pollutant levels. The air quality data provided does indicate that the Air Quality Control Region does not meet the National Air Quality Standards for particulates, SO_2, ozone, and CO at the present time. The prevailing winds in the area of the proposed plant site are predominantly from the south in the summer months. A major fossil-fuel power plant that burns high-sulfur coal is located 8 miles to the south of the proposed plant. During the winter the winds are from the northwest. More monitoring data is needed to determine the effects of a major metropolitan area located to the northwest of the site. This area is heavily industrialized, the largest industries being primary and fabricated metals, chemicals, and oil refining. Meaningful dispersion estimates could not be made because of the lack of emission and design information.

The need for characterization of the quantities and types of emissions from the plant, as a first step in the assessment of the potential threat to human health, is strongly indicated in light of the following information provided in the EAR:

1. Prevailing winds from the direction of the major point and area sources.
2. An annual average inversion frequency of 36%.
3. An annual average fog frequency of 10%.

Water

Water quality data were reported from two public agencies as well as some on-site testing. The testing was conducted one day in each of the months of September, November, and December, and so it cannot represent water quality changes throughout the year or give yearly averages. No sampling times or frequencies for the agency data were given. The data indicated that the river to be used as the receiving water for the proposed plant effluent already exceeds the Illinois State Water Quality Standards for phenol, iron, and manganese. Organic contaminants were found in fish from the river in one instance. However, it is unclear how much sampling was done for organic contaminants in aquatic organisms. In addition, ground water at the site, already disturbed by strip-mining, has been found to exceed the standard for total dissolved solids and iron.

The river serves as the major source of potable water for a town located downstream from the proposed plant. In addition, the river is stated to be a major source of recreation, chiefly boating and fishing, for the county. It is impossible to estimate the effect on the river quality from available data for the proposed plant. The already existing standard violations and possibility of agricultural and strip-mined land drainage indicate that very strict controls will be needed on the water effluent in order to protect the health of those using this resource.

Population Data

Extensive compilations of the population data in the counties surrounding the proposed plant were included in the report. Some breakdown on a countywide basis was made with regard to age, sex, and race. The purpose of including much of these data was unclear. Locations of schools, day-care centers, and nursing homes were not determined. The number of hospitals in the major communities was listed, but the locations were not given. No estimates for the number of chronically ill were made.

Correlation of the location of highest population densities and pollutant dispersion estimates was not done. The location of the most susceptible groups, children and elderly, was done on too broad a basis for population exposures to be made even if accurate pollutant dispersion estimates were possible. The possibility of health effects to the residents in the vicinity of the plant were summarized as follows: ''Contaminant concentrations are not likely to create any adverse impact outside of the site area because of their projected low levels'' (23). However, this statement contradicted earlier statements in the report that projections of these concentrations cannot be made. Occupational health was not addressed in the report.

SUMMARY

The Environmental Analysis Report discussed here was prepared as a preliminary document by which the decision could be made whether or not to prepare a full Environmental Impact Statement. Our evaluation provided a method to point out those areas that were lacking and the information still needed for a comprehensive and worthwhile Impact Statement. Although our analysis was necessarily incomplete, the approach did supply the basis for asking the right questions so that a rational evaluation could be carried out.

REFERENCES

1. U.S. Department of the Interior. *Energy Perspectives*. I 1.2:EN 2/6, 1975.
2. Federal Energy Administration. *National Energy Outlook, 1976, Executive Summary*. 1976.
3. Wadden, R. A. Coal hydrogenation and environmental health. *Environ. Health Perspect*. **14**:201–206, 1976.
4. Cooke, R. and Graham, P. W. The biological purification of the effluent from the Lurgi plant gasifying bituminous coals. *Int. J. Water Pollut*. **9**:97–112, 1965.
5. Forney, A. J., Haynes, W. P., Gasior, S. J., Johnson, G. E., and Strakey, J. P., Jr. *Analysis of Tars, Chars, Gases, and Water Found in Effluents from the Synthane Process*. Bureau of Mines Technical Progress Report, TPR 76, January 1974.
6. Ketcham, N. H. and Norton, R. W. The hazards to health in the hydrogenation of coal. III. The industrial hygiene studies. *Arch. Environ. Health* **1**:194–207, 1960.
7. Moeller, F. W., Roberts, H., and Britz, B. Methanation of coal gas for SNG. *Hydrocarbon Process*. **53**:69–91, 1974.
8. Sexton, R. J. The hazards to health in the hydrogenation of coal. I. An introductory statement on general information, process description, and a definition of the problem. *Arch. Environ. Health* **1**:181–186, 1960.
9. Attari, A., Pau, J., and Mensinger, M. *Fate of Trace and Minor Constituents of Coal During Gasification*. Environmental Protection Agency Report EPA-600/2-76-258, 1976.
10. World Health Organization. *Health Hazards of the Human Environment*. WHO, Geneva, 1972.
11. Donath, E. E. Hydrogenation of coal and tar. In *Chemistry of Coal Utilization* (Supplementary Volume). H. H. Lowry (Ed.). John Wiley & Sons, Inc., New York, 1963, p. 1041.
12. American Conference of Governmental Industrial Hygienists. *Documentation of the Threshold Limit Values*. ACGIH, Cincinnati, 1970, p. 180.
13. Ricketts, T. S. Modern methods of gas manufacture including the Lurgi process. *J. Inst. Fuel* **37**:328, 1964.
14. LeRoy, A. F. Interactions of platinum metals and their complexes in biological systems. *Environ. Health Perspect*. **10**:73–83, 1975.
15. Roberts, A. E. Platinosis. *Arch. Ind. Hyg*. **4**:549–559, 1951.
16. Weil, C. S. and Condra, N. I. The hazards to health in the hydrogenation of coal. II. Carcinogenic effect of materials on the skin of mice. *Arch. Environ. Health* **1**:187–193, 1960.
17. Seglin, L. and Eddinger, R. T. Coal (to synthetic crude oil). In *Encyclopedia of Chemical Technology Supplement*. R. E. Kirk and D. F. Othmer (Eds.), Interscience, New York, 1971, p. 195.

18. Sexton, R. J. The hazards to health in the hydrogenation of coal. IV. The control program and the clinical effects. *Arch. Environ. Health* **1**:208–231, 1960.

19. National Academy of Sciences. *Particulate Polycyclic Organic Matter.* Washington, DC, 1972.

20. Doll, R., Fisher, R. E. W., Gammon, E. J., Gunn, E., Hughes, G. O., Tyrer, F. H., and Wilson, W. Mortality of gasworkers with special reference to cancers of the lung and bladder, chronic bronchitis, and pneumoconiosis. *Br. J. Ind. Med.* **22**:1–12, 1965.

21. Lloyd, J. W. Long-term mortality study of steelworkers. V. Respiratory cancer in coke plant workers. *J. Occup. Med.* **13**:53–68, 1971.

22. Mazumdar, S., Redmond, C., Sollecito, W., and Sussman, N. An epidemiological study of exposure to coal tar pitch volatiles among coke oven workers. *J. Air Pollut. Control Assoc.* **25**:382–389, 1975.

23. Weston Environmental Consultants. *Coalcon Environmental Analysis Report, Vol. I and II.* Prepared for Energy Research and Development Administration, 1976.

24. U.S. Environmental Protection Agency, *Federal Regist.* **39**:42510, December 5, 1974.

INDEX